Also by Cari Corbet-Owen
The Mind over Fatter programme
ISBN: 1-919833-64-1

If you've tried the diets, bought the pills, read the books and still your weight yo-yo's - then Mind over Fatter is *the* non-diet plan for you. Say 'goodbye' to fatness and 'hello' to mental fitness. **(Ellen Hodgson Brown author of 11 published books including Nature's Pharmacy.)**

Many of us either never allow ourselves to get hungry or we're on some diet. Well, it's time to trust your body and its needs again. Mind Over Fatter provides realistic, back-to-basics tools by encouraging a truce between mind and body. It's a refreshingly sensible antidote to all the quick-fix prescriptive and restrictive diets out there. Consider it your personal, interactive textbook to healthy, permanent weight loss and self-love that's inspiring, motivating, and fun to read. **(SHAPE Magazine SA)**

Mind over Fatter gives you the knowledge, tips and tools to leave the diet rat race forever. It's the smartest Non-Diet, diet book around. **South African Nutrition Experts Panel (SANEP)**

The beauty of this book is that it's one you will go back to again and again. It is packed with information, ideas, snippets and wisdom that should have even the most dedicated food-obsessor wanting to break free from the tyranny of diet. **FITPREGNANCY Magazine (SA)**

In this (non-diet alternative) Mind over Fatter workbook, Cari Corbet-Owen expertly portrays the emotional underpinnings behind weight issues. This is done by making it clear that for those willing to engage in this holistic, self-healing and self-loving approach, it is 'never healthier to be self-hating than self-loving.' **ODYSSEY Magazine (SA)**

Have you struggled to lose weight and found yourself in an endless cycle of loss and regain? Are you tired of hating your body? Designed as a 'hands on' and practical approach to eating problems, this system is easy to use and understand…. This is more than just another diet plan, it is a profound system to change your life and self-image." **RENNAISANCE Magazine (SA)**

The

Joy-Filled

Body

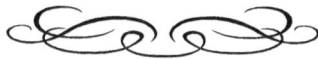

Cari Corbet-Owen
Clinical psychologist

Published by Joy-Filled Living

Napa, California

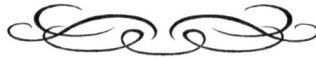

Text copyright: Cari Corbet-Owen (Clinical psychologist) 2008

This book has also been published under the title:
Mind over Fatter: Learn to feel great without ever dieting again
ISBN: 978 177020 0159
Oshun publishers 2007

ISBN: 978-0-6151-8896-6

Contents

Foreword
Acknowledgements
Preface
A glossary of terms
Disclaimer

Preface

The process of writing this book has amazed me. The way it has unfolded has felt at times as if its been orchestrated from a different level that has nothing to do with me, for the synchronicity of events that unfolded were more magical than anything I could ever have aspired to arranging. Three events in particular changed the entire shape of what you finally see on these pages.

The amazing Bev Bancroft, generously offered to start and be the moderator for our online Mind over Fatter support group from which so many of the wise morsels you will read have been drawn. It was uncanny how often I'd be working on a particular section only to have the group, start posting stories about the exact subject I was writing about.

Floris and Sebastian from Magical Dream Production, the company responsible for producing the Mind over Fatter DVD, asked me to watch "What the Bleep do we know" for ideas on how to produce our DVD. It provided me with unexpected but fascinating material.

Next, Napoleon Hill's book, "Think and grow rich" (which I've heard about for years but never felt inclined to read) fell into my hands. In it, he talks about holding mental meetings with people in order to help access their wisdom. This idea excited me – imagine if I could consult with great people to help me write this book! For not one minute did I realize when I sat quietly envisaging myself at a round table with five empty chairs and mentally 'inviting' whoever needed to be in the room to help me write this book and waited to see who would arrive, just how pivotal this process would be to writing this book. First through the 'door' was Nelson Mandela, next Oprah Winfrey, then the Dalai Lama followed by Leonardo Buscaglia and Dr. Wayne Dyer. Wow – these were all people I was in awe of and thrilled to have on 'my writing team.' However the composition surprised me, because with the exception of Oprah, I wondered what they knew about dieting and body. But I assumed they were the people who were meant to be there and once we were all 'seated,' I asked them: "What do I need to do to make this a great book?" To give you an idea of their incredible input, these are the 'minutes' taken from just our first two meetings:

Monday, August 07, 2006
Nelson: It's about releasing people from a mental prison. Remember my book: Long road to Freedom – this is no quick fix – you need to emphasize that this is a journey of the mind and not the body.
Oprah: It's got to be authentic, use real people's stories and don't forget to incorporate other authors whose wisdom you've internalized.
Dalai Lama: It's about freeing people from oppression
Leonardo: The key to releasing people from oppression and mental prisons is self-love
Wayne: Tell them about the spiritual journey –it's not the body that's important but their soul they need to give emphasis to. Remind them that when they're too focused on the exterior it takes their focus from their greater purpose.

Wednesday, August 09, 2006
Agenda: on releasing people from mental prisons
Nelson: you have to show them how prisons are mental. Even though I was jailed, I wouldn't allow them to jail my mind. I looked passed the bars to see all the possibilities rather than into the bars and all the restrictions.
Oprah: Don't trap yourself into an impossible dream. Rather change your dream than be trapped in one that keeps you in jail.
Dalai Lama: remember the story about the Buddhist whose house burn down and the remedy was laughter. Houses aren't meant to burn down, and you aren't meant to laugh if they do. Well bodies apparently aren't meant to grow large and you aren't meant to laugh if they do – but you can change that.
Leonardo: Nobody hugs those poor bars, everyone avoids them and hates them – it's no wonder they stay all firm and rigid. Take the thoughts that form your prison bars and hug them…. Kill them with kindness so they can dissolve through the force of love alone.
Wayne: Remember Ivangeli…. She was trapped in a physical prison, but she never allowed that to imprison her hopes and dreams. Instead she used this time to forge an even stronger connection with her Creator. Your body is like that physical prison, you can either allow it to imprison your hopes and dreams, or in spite of it you can force a stronger connection with your Creator. That choice is yours.
      And, as if those three events weren't pivotal enough, other things happened during the writing of this book that were simply miraculous. My web-browser opened on the 'wrong' webpage (not once but three times), providing me with incredible research to support an idea that had just popped into my head. I 'forgot' to take a book on a weekend away and the book that falls into my hands instead: Power vs. Force is an important work for this

book. Candace Pert's book, All you need to know Go(o)d fell onto my foot during a visit to a bookstore. Like I said, there was a power far greater than myself involved in the writing of this book. Without this Greater Power, I, alone, could not possibly have come up with what appears on the pages of this book.

Acknowledgements

I'd like to acknowledge every Mind over Fatter body pilgrim I have ever worked with throughout the years, especially my online 'family.' Their painful dieting stories and their wisdom when it comes to leaving the yo-yo diet bandwagon continue to inspire me. I am forever indebted to their generosity when it comes to allowing me to share their enormous knowledge about their bodies, food, eating and recovery. While Mind over Fatter might be 'my' baby, it really isn't 'mine' - because it's a collection or many people's wisdom. It's a bit like Mind over Fatter is a body. It has some bones (the wonderful people I work with), some flesh (the course material), but the muscle is the Mind over Fatter body pilgrims – without them it would have no life. It's grown too big for me to breathe life into all on my own. Without the Mind over Fatter family who keep it alive with their morsels of wisdom, it would get anorexia and die.

I would like to thank my mental advisors: Nelson Mandela, Oprah Winfrey, The Dalai Lama, Leonardo Buscaglia and Dr. Wayne Dyer. In so many ways, they are all co-authors to this book. In addition, the ideas of many other authors have also been incorporated into this text, however as it has often become internalized, I'm not always able to remember how a certain bit of information came to be a part of my thinking. I'd also like to thank Joanne Ikeda for meeting with me and providing me with research that took my old ingrained thinking and opened me up to new possibilities which form the central core of this book. Dr. David Hawkins, author of Power vs. Force graciously read sections of this book and gave me the thumbs up saying this book was "good work" – thanks to him for taking time out of his busy schedule to do this.

Glossary of terms used

Diet City: A place of the mind where living in your body is painful and filled with thoughts of not being good enough and restlessly attempting any- and everything to change it.

Nature's Valley: A place of the mind where you are in like with yourself and where you trust and respect your body's ability to self-regulate. Food, exercise and your body are a joy instead of something to fear.

Thinland: A place of smoke and mirrors within the mind where you live in the belief that being thin will miraculously solve every problem you have.

Body pilgrim: a person on the Mind over Fatter journey from Diet City back to Nature's Valey

Food Jail: A place of the mind where you're trapped in calorie-counting, worrying about whether what you're eating is 'legal' or 'illegal', or just being hypervigilent and uncomfortable around food.

Psychological hooks: Subconscious snares your mind sets up to keep you hooked into old attitudes and habits.

Deep Essential truths: Values that are enduring and empowering and don't change historically or from one culture to the next.

Surface ego beliefs: Values that are unstable, that change over time or in different cultures.

Epigraph

Throughout *The Joy-Filled Body*, you'll hear me talking about the Mind over Fatter which is an emotional, physical and spiritual HEALTH-GAIN program. It's a program about getting your MIND over this whole 'fatter' issue. And of course it does contain fabulous guidelines for eating and exercising naturally (and healthily), however, its goal is not thinness. Weight loss is merely a by-product of health-gain. The program's goal is to allow you to live in a joy-filled body without all the angst about food, eating, exercising and dieting. With this in mind pilgrims achieve different things on the Mind over Fatter program as these morsels below show. **This book, *The Joy-Filled Body* is the logical follow-on step after Mind over Fatter although the benefits of reading it even without having read Mind over Fatter are in no way diminished.**

I haven't lost any weight (gave that up years ago!!) , exercise keeps me as I am, which is heavier/higher body fat percentage than one would expect for the type of things I have done for fun. Have climbed Kilimanjaro ran a race across the Kalahari Desert and this year ran across The Alps (240km in 8 days, through 4 countries), raising R50 000 for The Smile Foundation in the process.

I can't remember where I first heard about Mind over Fatter but years ago I read the book/programme and certain things stuck in my head, like seeing exercise as 'body fun' and not as an arduous task that one should do just to keep healthy or to lose weight. I have always enjoyed sport, especially at school and University, but when I decided that I needed to lose weight after my three children had been born, I found myself considering exercise as purely a means to an end - that perfect figure (that will never be!!) and it was at times almost a punishment, especially gym sessions. Even though I've always loved running (ran marathons in my 20's), at times I would get out onto the road just to burn up calories, which also felt like punishment. Understanding the Mind over Fatter philosophy has changed that - I now see it as fun, good for my body and mind, and a great way to meet people and see new places. And if I do a weights session I view it as an accompaniment to my running training, to increase my strength endurance. All a matter of attitude I suppose! (Jan: November, 23rd, 2007)

My name is Joy and I began this journey in Sept 2004. I embarked on "Project Joy" getting my head together, doing the Mind over Fatter emotional processing workshops, had therapy and all of that good stuff in preparation for the radical re-emergence of ME! At the time I weighed 187kg (411lbs), which on a 7ft frame is not attractive, so on my measly 1.52m (5ft) it looked positively monstrous! Since then I have managed to reshape myself into a rounded 69kg (151lbs) without being on a diet (and yes I think I am positively miniscule!) It's been a hard road not because I have been on a "diet" but because I have had to ask and answer (and am still asking and trying to answer!) all the big/hard/real questions. The real challenge for me has been in redefining all my relationships - from my marriage to children, friends and siblings. .It is a process as much around how you reshape your thinking as your body. And this is necessary for sustainability. . It's been a physical, emotional and spiritual journey or re-discovery. (Joy: October 11, 2006)

Lets face it what we need is a healthy mind in a healthy body. If it wasn't for Mind over Fatter, my goal in life wouldn't have been a fit and healthy body, it would have been to be skinny. And that is SO NOT what its all about!! We don't measure our progress in kilos and centimetres. We measure it in our degrees to which our thinking has changed about our bodies, food, weight etc. .....this is a journey of acceptance and realising self worth. And definitely not a quick fix! (Marelise: November 28th, 2007)

To the people in my life who encourage my inner child to come out and play: My husband Corby, my parents Geoff and Lynn Harris, my siblings Brett, Bev and Lara, my special friend the LYH, and the special and amazing children in my life: Amy, Shannon, Sarah-Kate, Ross and Troy.

Disclaimer

Other than the stories of Jane, Joy and Marelise, the story-morsels I have shared here carry no names or biographical details. Every morsel comes from my many dealings with pilgrims engaged in the struggle of leaving Diet City be they during individual therapy session, group workshops, radio- or TV program phone-ins. Many morsels have been harvested from online support groups – most particularly the Mind over Fatter online community (mindoverfatter-subscribe@yahoogroups.com). Almost every morsel has been edited for brevity and often grammar, or I may have combined two parts of a person's conversation, however I've endeavoured to ensure their original meaning stays accurate. I am aware that many Mind over Fatter pilgrims whose smatterings of wisdom are to be found on these pages will read what they have said and find themselves in a different stage of their journey. Some will look on their words, reflect on how they have changed and grown and be pleased with their progress. Others will believe they have regressed, and feel bad that they have let me or Mind over Fatter down. Fortunately neither would be true, Mind over Fatter doesn't happen in a straight line, backwards and forwardsing, ups and downs are all just an expected part of the journey.

Chapter 1

♥

Introduction

Whatever happened to the times when our bodies were a source of fun and enjoyment? Where did they go, those carefree times of childhood, when food wasn't an issue, when we weren't at war with our bodies, and when play and laughter ruled our lives rather than the scale, our clothes size or our latest diet? When did listening to our bodies disappear, along with appreciating the simple joy of food, dancing with carefree abandon and loving every bit of ourselves?

Fact is, neither naturally thin people nor young children live balanced on a tightrope of self-deprecation, restrictive dieting and deprivation in order to stay slender. So what's their secret?

The answers are astonishingly logical and simple. *The Joy-Filled Body* offers you glimpses of a future where a return to a great attitude towards food and your body is not just possible, but also probable. It's a journey that offers respite and liberation to people who are sick and tired of the same old diet bandwagon with its never-ending but forever failing mutations.

The Joy-Filled Body journey has as its destination a 'state of mind and of being' rather than a 'state of body'. And the constant guiding principles are LOVE and JOY. At each crossroad, we need only ask ourselves: "What step do I need to take in order to become more self-loving and to fall more deeply in love with life?" It's not about needing to relearn new behaviour, but about letting go of erroneous beliefs about our body so that our inner wisdom can once more be revealed to us. We *all* have the inner power and wisdom we need to transform our bodies and minds back into the joy- and peace-filled state they once were – it's just waiting to be rediscovered.

We can't get there, though, if we're stuck in the harsh 'giraffe syndrome'. A baby giraffe has no sooner fallen a few metres from its mother's womb when the mother kicks it repeatedly until it wobbles back onto its legs. If it falls, the mother kicks it again and the baby giraffe has to repeat the struggle in order to build its leg strength so it can keep up with the herd.

Isn't this exactly what we do to ourselves when it comes to dieting? You kick yourself when you're down, when the latest diet has failed you. It's this process that keeps you trapped within that herd following the diet industry – the belief that it's essential to get up and try yet another diet.

This kicking may well keep baby giraffes safe from predators but, sadly, it only keeps diets preying on us. So long as the billion-dollar diet industry can con us into believing that *we* are the failures and not their (usually expensive) product, they're always going to have the upper hand. Well, the simple fact is that if their products were as wonderful as they would have us believe, the world's weight problems would be over by now. We need to realize *we* aren't failing; its diets that fail us!

I have labelled the 'place' (state of mind) where naturally slim people and many children live Nature's Valley, but sadly most of us have migrated from it over the years, so that our minds (and often our bodies as well) now reside in Diet City. This is a 'place' where we are either:

- on diet,
- considering dieting,
- worried about gaining the extra weight we might never even had or the weight we have just lost,
- just plainly obsessing about food and eating,
- finding activity to be a bore or a chore, or
- living in dislike or disharmony with our bodies.

If you are experiencing any of these, you are a resident of Diet City: a Dietonian.

Diet City is a haphazard and confusing maze of conflicting (mis)information. Its garbage site is piled high with empty promises, failed diets, unused gym contracts, discarded home exercise machines, guilt, shame, hopelessness and despair. Every diet promises it will lead you to that utopia known as Thinland, the 'place' where you will finally be truly happy. Problem is, Thinland is just another cul-de-sac. If you're still obsessing about food, eating, exercising and your weight and/or shape, I don't care how thin you are, you're still trapped in Diet City. *The Joy-Filled Body* is a journey out of Diet City and back to the contented 'place' of Nature's Valley.

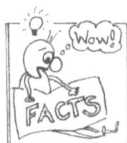

I'd rather die than be fat!
A large online sample of 4283 respondents, 46% said they would rather give up one year of life than be obese, and 30% reported that they would rather be divorced than be obese.

2

And here's typical Dietonian thinking: in each case, *thinner* people were more willing to sacrifice aspects of their health or life circumstances than the heavier people. Normal, healthy people have been terrorised into fearing fat! [1]

The four-letter D-word

Why is the Western world getting fatter and unhealthier? Sure, we have fast-food joints popping up like flowers in spring, but the same can be said for health food stores and fat-free, sugar-free products. We might well have more TVs, drive everywhere in our cars and take escalators and lifts instead of walking up the stairs, but we also have gyms and health clubs opening left, right and centre. Dietonians spend whopping – and ever-increasing – amounts on diet products, so you'd assume they'd be getting thinner and not fatter, right? Wrong! There is an alarming corresponding rise in obesity (and eating disorders).

A lot focus is given out there to the physical elements theoretically influencing weight gain – eating and exercise. But after 15 years of scouring thousands of medical and psychological journals, I've come to the conclusion that there are other factors that no-one seems to take into account. And one is that four-letter D-word! Diets wreak havoc on your body – not only physically, but mentally and emotionally too. Diets also make you fatter.

Diets have 'illegal', foods which is a fabulous way to trigger cravings for those very foods which easily spirals you out of control. It is dieting that starts the vicious cycle. You eat something that you classify as illegal, next comes the guilt followed by even more eating to stuff down those feelings of failure. You begin body-bashing and hating yourself, and, eventually, with help form the diet industry, you convince yourself that *you're* the problem. Allowing a diet to control what, how and when you eat plays a pivotal role in creating unhealthy dieting patterns. Dieting is not the *only* factor involved, but there's certainly no denying that it plays a much bigger role than the diet industry would ever admit to.

The stress of dieting

Living in a larger body than our Western culture dictates is frowned upon in a very public way - 'fatism' is alive and well. [2] Its one of the few prejudices that is openly practised in the way of rude comments and fat jokes. The result? Being forced to live in Diet City, which is to live in a constant state of un-love, anxiety and fear.

3

Tomes of research give evidence that supports the role *stress* plays in causing disease and health problems. Stress exacerbates all health conditions (for example, cardiovascular problems, hypertension and type II diabetes), which, we are constantly told, are caused by being overweight. So, take a deep breath, because I want to pose a question that has mind-spinning ramifications: What if many of the health challenges fatties face come about more because of the ongoing, unacknowledged tension that accompanies living in a body constantly criticised by ourselves (and others) – rather than the weight itself? *What if it were true that many of the health problems that appear to be so prevalent are caused (or severely exacerbated) by living continually in a harsh emotional space and by us not being self-loving enough? And what about how our beliefs about our health affect our bodies?*

Those questions probably raised a cacophony of protestations: I can just hear the prevalent Diet city thinking: 'But being unhappy with my body is a *good* thing because body dissatisfaction is what it takes in order for me to *do* something about it, right?' Wrong! The problem is, we *do* do something about it (even the skinnies amongst us). We diet. We get thinner, fatter, we diet again, get thinner – but not as thin as we were before – then get fatter, and even fatter. We diet again… See the problem? [3]

Diets only work for up to 5% of people in the long-term. What a spectacular failure rate! If any other specific health or medical product had such a dismal track record, it would have been ditched years ago. How many diabetics would still be taking medication if it meant their sugar levels improved in the short term but ultimately got worse for 95% of them in the long term? What if the *medication* was in fact *worsening* their condition in the long term? [4]

For the vast majority, not only do fad diets definitely *not* maintain weight loss but Dietonians worldwide weigh *more* the more they've dieted. Here's why: with each fad-lose-it-fast-diet you lose healthy muscle and water only to gain back unhealthy fat because, in the process, your body slows it's metabolism (to conserve energy) and store fat more efficiently (for when you need that energy, since fat is a source of energy). Not only does the supposed cure for being fat *not* achieve what it boasts it does, but diets play a major role in *causing* the very thing they supposedly prevent!

And we haven't even touched on the effects that health-eroding repeated losses and gains have on our self-confidence. If you're one of those dedicated Dietonians who has been there, done that and only got the stretch marks, xxxl t-shirts and feeling of failure to show for it, then you'll know this. Even though diets don't work, the pressure to diet is constant, and it often comes from those closest to us.

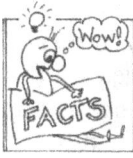

Research was done in 2006 at Yale University on 2671 overweight and obese adults in terms of how they coped when they were exposed to anti-fat attitudes. These overweight adults reported that physicians and family members were the ones who most frequently commented negatively on their weight. Also, people who had begun dieting earlier in life reported more stigmatising situations than people who started dieting later. *The earlier we start and the harder we try to lose weight by dieting, the more anti-fat prejudice we encounter and the more stress society places on us.*

The study also looked at coping mechanisms these adults used to deal with the negative attitudes of those around them. Here's the kicker: number four on a list of coping strategies was ... eating! So let me emphasise this point: Those well-meaning family members and medical professionals, often the very people instrumental in our earliest dieting efforts and who keep harping on about our weight, are unwittingly promoting comfort eating – the very thing they're doing their best to make us avoid!

Does this story sound familiar? *I'd lost 33lbs and my mom came to visit. She didn't notice (argh!) and then kindly gave me a top she'd bought me with the words: 'I think it'll fit because it's a big size'! Whenever I came back from college she would feed me for a few days – then one day, when I reached for a piece of her cake, she'd suddenly say: 'Do you really think you should, dear?'* Before long these subtle comments become part of our own thoughts, and that's when the real damage occurs. In the next chapter, we discuss the impact that negative self-thoughts have physically (in scientifically measurable ways) on our health and well-being.

You *can* be too thin

As much of the world becomes more obese, there's also been an alarming increase in people with other kinds of eating disorders. These, too, develop from a space of self-criticism. *I developed OCD (obsessive compulsive disorder). I would do 'mirror work' (which involves finely inspecting your body) all day every day. I would beat myself up about eating just one chocolate, I would binge and take laxatives, and I would binge and vomit. I was totally out of control.*

As a psychologist with a special interest in this field, I cannot help but notice that the variety of eating disorders has burgeoned – from anorexia and bulimia to now include binge-eating disorder (eating large quantities), night-eating disorder, orthorexia (overzealous healthy eating), bigorexia (an obsession with muscle-toning) and exercise bulimia (using exercise as a compensatory measure). Although not all of these are classified as official eating disorders, their existence shows just how painfully complex our relationships with food and our bodies are becoming. Added to this, the age range of those affected by eating disorders has increased. In March 2007 a BBC report cited a six-year-old with anorexia and I've worked with a woman in her late sixties who had bulimia. Eating disorders now affect men as well as previously unaffected ethnic groups and geographical regions. In Fiji, when commercial TV arrived in 1995, it only took three years for 12% of Fijian teens to develop an eating disorder. [5]

It's no secret that our attempts to lose weight are often the swiftest route to eating disorders. Consider this: bulimia sufferers are almost always dieters turned bingers turned purgers in a crazy attempt to meet the 'body beautiful' criteria. Anorexia victims are just on a protracted diet of obsessively restrictive eating and/or exercising to become thin. And those of us who belong to slimming clubs binge-eat more than overweight women who aren't members. [6] But hear this: you don't find eating disorders in naturalist villages and culture where large bodies are thought of as beautiful!

We need to stop listening to this never-ending call to lose weight. Fad diets lead to weight-gain and poorer health. When we only focus on looking thinner, we aren't necessarily gaining health and we aren't necessarily gaining joy of self-love either. We could in fact be gaining thinness and, ironically, *losing* health! A thinner you isn't *always* healthier and a fatter you isn't *always* unhealthier either.

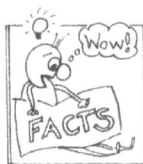

Fat is bad, thin is good?
Scientists in Denmark found that the survival rates of 13 000 patients with blood clots, heart disease and brain haemorrhages increased proportionally up to a body mass index (divide your weight in kilograms by the square of your height in meters) of 35. Being that 27 is the BMI level at which we are apparently obese, this flies in the face of what we have been taught to believe: fat is bad, thin is good. That is not always true as a growing amount of research is proving and at any rate, it is way too simplistic. [6a]

For example, a startling new study of 2.3 million Americans published by the respected Nov 2007 edition of the Journal of the American Medical Association has caused consternation among public health professionals. It's originates not from some fast food chain or fringe group of scientists but rather from the analysis of decades of data by federal researchers at the Centres for Disease Control and Prevention (CDC) in Atlanta, Georgia. Its conclusion supports that found by Danish and other Scandinavian researchers: carrying a little extra weight appears to be beneficial for your health and may help people to live longer. Dr. Elizabeth Barrett-Connor, professor of family and preventive medicine at the University of California, San Diego, agrees with the studies findings because she believes that a BMI of 25 to 30 - roughly the so-called overweight range - "may be optimal." The bottom line, scientists say, is that modestly overweight people demonstrate a lower death rate than their peers who are underweight, obese or – most surprisingly – 'normal weight. Those Americans who were merely overweight were up to about 40 per cent less likely than normal-weight people to die from a whole range of diseases and risks including emphysema, pneumonia, Alzheimer's, injuries and various infections. Aside from escaping diseases, Dr Flegal, the lead researcher in this study says that having more bodily reserves also helps people recover from serious surgery, injuries and infections, so they have more to draw on in times of medical crisis.[6b]

The media constantly harp about the hazards of obesity but we don't seem to see, front-cover news about the dangers of very low-calorie diets that have high death rates. Nor do we hear how dangerous the inevitable rapid fat regain after dieting is.

And before I'm sliced, diced and popped into a blender, I'm not disputing that weight loss results mostly in improvements in many areas of health. But when your inevitable weight regain follows, all your health indices quickly return to where they were, often *surpassing* their previously unhealthy levels – even after only a fraction of your weight loss has been regained. Our yo-yoing weight losses and gains double our chances of dying from cardiovascular disease [8], the greatest cause of death for women. How many of us actually realize it is vastly healthier to gradually gain weight than to seesaw?

Let's face it: the diet industry has a lot to answer for with its never-ending supply of gee-whiz cure-alls for weight problems. But, given that they don't work, are there natural alternatives? And, more importantly, are we prepared to hear them?

Health At Every Size (HAES)

Some health professionals, faced with the rising prevalence of obesity, the dismal track record of dieting and the premise that obesity may actually be relatively benign when compared with dieting habits themselves, have begun to suspect that believing in diets is like still believing the world is flat. This is good because it finally frees up resources to start researching new paradigms – such as the relatively new idea that we can be healthy at any size. Professor Linda Bacon, who conducted a two-year study into dieting versus no dieting at the University of California, says: 'We have been ingrained to think that seriously large people can only make improvements in their health if they diet and slim down. But this study tells us that you can make significant improvements in both metabolic and psychological health without ever stepping on the scales or counting calories. You can relax about food.' [9]

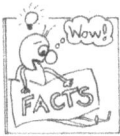

This important study comprised of a dieting group (dieters) and a non-dieting group (non-dieters) who followed the Health at Every Size (HAES) model. The HAES model focuses not on monitoring food intake but instead trains participants to pay more attention to internal body cues that signal hunger and fullness. Dieters moderately restricted their food consumption, monitored their weight and kept food diaries. They were counselled about the benefits of exercise, behavioural strategies for successful dieting, calorie counting and fat content, reading food labels and appropriate food-shopping. Non-dieters replaced their restrictive eating habits with paying attention to internal body cues. They were counselled about becoming more accepting of their larger bodies, healthy food choices, identifying and dealing with barriers that might get in the way of enjoying physical activity and they also learned how culture influences the experience of obese people.

What Dr. Bacon and her researchers found is impressive!

- ♥ 92% of the non-dieting group compared to 42% of the dieting group completed the study. Doesn't that just prove how unsustainable diets are?
- ♥ Dieters initially lost 5.2% of their weight but regained almost all of it back by the end of the two-year study period. Non-dieters' weight stayed the same throughout the study. They at least didn't have the fat regain and one more dent to their self-confidence to deal with.

- ♥ Dieters showed no significant change in cholesterol levels throughout the study whereas the non-dieters had an initial increase in their total cholesterol levels which then decreased significantly (including LDL, or 'bad' cholesterol) by the end of the study.
- ♥ Both groups significantly lowered their systolic blood pressure which was sustained by the non-dieters but not the dieters.
- ♥ By the end of the study, non-dieters had almost quadrupled their physical activity whereas the dieters who increased their physical activity had slipped back to their initial levels by the end of the study.
- ♥ Non-dieters demonstrated significant improvements in self-esteem and depression by the end the study, while dieters' self-esteem levels had worsened.

The conclusion?

Non-dieters may not have lost significant weight, but they'd nevertheless succeeded in improving their overall health, as measured by cholesterol levels, blood pressure, physical activity and self-esteem.

Any improvements made by the diet group were not sustained and their self-esteem had plummeted. Need I say more? This is so typical of dieting.

Is fat really the big health ogre?
In Europe, many studies have been done on whether it is in fact unhealthy to be fat. The results are fascinating.

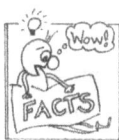

In a research study in 2003 comparing groups from Denmark and Greenland, the Inuit population of Greenland had lower levels of glucose and insulin, blood pressure, and triglycerides, and higher levels of HDL ('good' cholesterol) than the Danish participants *at any given level of obesity*. [10] No matter what the level of obesity, the Inuit's' health indicators were always better than those of the Danes, *so level of fatness wasn't what made the difference*. Additionally, a study of middle-aged Swedish women found that the death rate *fell* steadily with increasing fatness, even at the upper extremes of obesity. [11] In an enormous study of 1.8 million Norwegians over 10 years, the highest death rate occurred in underweight women and the lowest mortality rate of all was amongst those who were approximately 30% overweight. (Hold on... isn't this the level at which we're told we're obese and unhealthy?) Even women considered 'morbidly obese' had lower death rates than the underweight group. [12] Another study based on the evidence from this Norwegian study divided the women into four groups: the skinnies, the 'insurance ideal', the overweight and the morbidly obese, then predicted their life expectancy. The skinniest group – the cultural icon of beauty (the equivalent of 5ft6 in height, weighing 109lbs) – had the shortest life expectancy with only 730 women in 1000 living to age 65. In the group where the women weighed what the height-versus-weight chart indicated she should, 824 women in 1000 would live to age 65. Surprisingly, of those who were considered overweight (5ft6 tall, weighing 224lbs), 844 were predicted to reach age 65 – the highest life expectancy. And even the 'morbidly obese' group (weighing in at over 279lbs) outlived the skinny model group with 757 in 1000 expected to make it to age 65. [13]

Of the many factors that affect health, extra weight may not be the worst of them. How many health professionals (and I'm including my colleagues, because not only are we often major culprits in perpetuating the diet myth and fat prejudices, but we are also able to have a powerful impact on correcting misinformation) know that diets *exacerbate* the situation and that being overweight isn't always the heinous health hazard it's made out to be? A colleague once told me: *I'm part of the health industry, but from where I was looking for many years, it seemed more like the 'skinny at all costs' industry. If health followed as an added bonus, great.* Well, *The Joy-Filled Body* wants to help you to feel healthy – physically, mentally and emotionally. And striving to be skinny isn't how to go about it. Striving to live in a joy-filled body is.

What works for you?

Suggesting that we need to diet down to the cultural ideas of thinness is an invitation to frustration and added stress. What we *don't* need is body hatred and dieting. What we *do* need instead is acceptance and encouragement to follow a healthy, active and self-loving lifestyle.

Diet products and eating plans don't honour your uniqueness or your unique lifestyle and needs. They don't take into account that your body is not simply skin, bones, muscle and adipose tissue but also fields of information, intelligence and energy. They don't emphasise the importance of personal growth, nor do they tell you that for each pound you lose, you should work on gaining self-love. They pretend the journey to feeling comfortable in your body is a simple linear event where you go from 'being bad' (not watching what you eat) to apparently 'being good' (sticking to yet another unnatural and unsustainable way to lose weight). They don't tell you that it's often in wandering off the track or sometimes looking at your life and situation from an upside-down or inside-out perspective that you find out more about your wonderful self and what works for you.

The Joy-Filled Body is a journey of liberation that goes backwards in order to go forwards. The answers to living healthily, with love, lightness, laughter and a feeling of ease and comfort in your own skin, are to be found in your early childhood. They are to be found in the times before your 'love of self' and your wisdom about how to regulate your body naturally became eroded by cultural 'wisdom' and well-intentioned but misguided caregivers. Essentially, returning to Nature's Valley is about doing what you once did instinctively as young children: eating when you're hungry; loving to be active; feeling fine about seeing yourself in the mirror or photographs; and having fun as you live life. And the great news is that these morsels of wisdom I am sharing show a way to do this without being a slave to the scale, without restriction, deprivation, crazy eating plans, throwing up food, or being critical of you.

When it comes to feeling comfortable in your body, the overall goal of *The Joy-Filled Body* is to help you change the state of your mind and habits, but how you go about achieving it will vary. If you are a wife who has three children and works full-time, what will work for you is likely to be very different from what might work for a single working woman. If you were brought up in an abusive family, your issues with food and your body will need to be tackled differently from someone who also struggles with emotional eating yet comes from a warm and loving background. In sharing these morsels, my hope is that you will discover there is no single escape path from Diet City. Some of you may want to go at a relatively fast pace, others need only go as fast as the slowest part of you wishes to travel.

This book gives you valuable tips gleaned from the journeys of others who've also struggled to leave the maze of Diet City for the serenity of Nature's Valley. Their stories will help you realize that you are not alone on this journey. As you read each morsel, be open to the insight that a pilgrim's experience might provide you, enabling you to free yourself from even one small part of Diet City. Alternatively, their story may serve to highlight what isn't an issue for you.

And pssst ... here's the incredibly simple secret: returning to Nature's Valley 'is like that butterfly that keeps eluding you if you run after it, but comes and sits on your shoulder when you stop chasing it'. [14]

Chapter 2:

♥

Your Emotional Body

A 2006 post on 'Big Fat Blog' proclaimed: 'I'd rather be stupid and mean than fat.' How did this one three-lettered word get to carry so much weight? I'm quite sure no other three letters bear the weight of such judgement and criticism. *We are swimming in a sea of fat-hating, diet-pushing, money-grabbing nonsense.* It's difficult to remember just how Sacred and wondrous you are when you're so hating and disparaging of the body in which your Sacredness is hidden. I am sad for whoever penned these words. They speak volumes about the harshness of the inner critic that resides in his or her mind. Making this kind of harsh judgement isn't inherent in human nature; it's culturally imposed by a society that has forgotten we are *all* Sacred regardless of our appearance.

We're Sacred because, as Dr Wayne Dyer points out in *Your Sacred Self*, we are 'spiritual beings having a human experience rather than human beings having a spiritual one'. He explains this by saying, when we bite into a piece of apple pie, we don't expect it to taste like cherry or pineapple, because we know it comes from apples. Thus, if we originate from a Creator, then we must be 'a slice' of that Creator, not simply a bunch of cells fashioned into a body. If we were to form a body cast around ourselves and then remove it, it would be obvious that what the cast lacks is our essence, our spirit. If we acknowledge that we are a piece of our Creator, we can also acknowledge that the part of us that counts the most (our Essential Self) has God-like qualities – greatness, love and kindness. So when we forget we are Sacred beings, we in fact have Edged God Out – we have developed an EGO state. Thus the *whole* of you, including your body, is sacred, so any thoughts you might have that downgrade your body are an insult to your Creator. When you flip your thinking in this way, you being made in the Creator's image takes on a whole new meaning.

This way around, your body isn't the centre of everything; your soul is what's eternal and enduring. Your body is merely a temporary vessel. Deepak Chopra talks about the body being like a cloak you can just let fall to the floor when you die. And yet, we frantically fret about our bodies, trying to mould and panel-beat them into shape, forgetting they have a sell-by-date. In the process, the beauty of our souls gets pushed aside. But then advertisers haven't yet found a way to 'package' the soul to sell products. No single soul is more valuable or special than another, and prejudice against a person purely because his or her body doesn't meet some randomly imposed cultural standard should be outlawed.

Whoever typed those words on the Big Fat Blog wasn't speaking from his or her Essential Self, but rather his/her Ego Self. It's a bizarrely crazy notion that how we appear on the outside is more important than honouring the divinity inherent in each one of us. We've been conned into thinking it's our eating habits that are self-destructive, but what's *really* destructive is forgetting that we are deserving of love, no matter what, and then keeping harsh self-judgements alive in our hearts.

Let's face it; what we believe to be true isn't always The Truth. Once upon a time the earth really was believed to be flat and, incredibly, in the 1950s, doctors promoted smoking as a health practice. Research bias (that is, we find what we expect to be the truth, hence look for only that) is well documented. Once an idea has been established as '*the* truth,' researchers will find evidence that supports it over and over because they are blinded to other possibilities that don't fit into their current frame of reference. The questions asked by researchers – which give rise to answers they're looking for – as well as the way they examine and make their research data meaningful, are limited by the viewpoint they hold. For example: the Royal College of Physicians' official medical report in 1983 revealed that rural South Africans have a high prevalence of obesity without the expected morbidity and mortality. Had I been one of those researchers, I'm sure I would have been intrigued to have found this group that stood out from the norm, as my mindset at the time would have had me firmly convinced that fat people can only be unhealthy people. I'd probably have also concurred with their conclusions –it was environmental. The cause was their diet – low in fat and high in unrefined fibre-rich carbohydrates.

However, I started questioning a lot of what I've thought to be 'true' after meeting Dr Joanne Ikeda, a veteran nutrition education specialist of 30 years, from Berkeley University (California). She introduced me to an impressive body of research showing that fat people can be healthy when they're living a healthy lifestyle. Since then, additional new ideas I've been introduced to have surprised and excited me. Finally, I'm taking a few deep breaths myself and daring to ask some questions out loud.

But first, I'm not denying that the rural diet of black South Africans plays a role. I'm a great advocate for healthy eating and active lifestyles. Of course, another *big* factor is that these black South Africans haven't subjected themselves to all the harmful yo-yo diets. I should also point out that they walk everywhere and carry out manual labour for hours on end.

But with all the new ideas in my head, I'm wondering if there aren't other enormously powerful factors – like our internal biochemistry – that researchers might never have considered. However, in order to explain my thinking, I need you to accompany me into the rabbit hole of body image, the brain and Biochemistry 101.

Your body image

In the Western world, body image is big, *really* big in terms of how much it impacts our lives. In fact, Dr Thomas Cash in *The Body Image Workbook*, says that at least two-thirds of our self-image consists of our body image. In other words, what you believe about your body plays a huge role in whether you feel negative or positive about yourself. If you're a Dietonian you'll know that on 'good' body days, life's a breeze and your body flaws fade into the background. But on 'bad' body days it's easy to feel upset, hopeless, frustrated, and insecure and to have constant critical thoughts about you. And as I'm about to propose, *the emotions linked to your body image affect your physical body in scientifically measurable ways.*

Your brain

The power of the mind is truly amazing! I was paging through our caterers catalogue to order food for our year-end Christmas function, and just reading about the different dishes had me salivating and made me feel ravenous. I could literally smell and imagine the taste of the food, and there weren't even pictures, only typed pages of menus! Using scanning techniques, scientists have discovered that the brain cannot tell the difference between what is real and what is imagined as, under both conditions, exactly the same areas of the brain are activated. Thus, if you're angry, a certain part of the brain is activated; if you *imagine* an event that invokes the feelings of anger, exactly the same part of the brain is stimulated. And here's the important bit: *your body chemistry reacts exactly the same way in both the imagined and the real situation.*

Test this yourself. Place a slice of lemon on your tongue and notice what happens in your mouth. Then repeat this using only your imagination; imagine the cool feeling as the lemon slice lands on your tongue and 'taste' the immediately strong sour flavor. Notice what happens in your mouth.

In both instances, intracellular messengers race through our system, transmitting messages via our cells so that saliva (which aids digestion) is released into your mouth.

Your biochemistry

Basically, a thought creates an electrical impulse in a neuron which then travels in a step-by-step sequence but with lightning-speed down the length of the cell until it reaches the small gap (a synapse) between that cell and the next. Here this electrical impulse sets off a chemical reaction so that small neurotransmitter-containing sacs open, vibrating their chemicals into the gap. These chemicals float over to the second cell and attach themselves to receptor sites there. Once enough of the receptor sites on the second cell are filled, another electrical impulse is generated, which travels down this next cell until it reaches the next synapse. This process is repeated over and over, cascading chemical messages across our cellular network, changing our endocrine, neurological, gastrointestinal, immune and other body systems. This intracellular communication, allows a high-speed transfer of information, throughout the entire body.

How you becoming emotionally addicted

When this process is repeated persistently, according to Canadian neurophysiologist Donald Hebb [15], some growth process or metabolic change takes place so that the firing becomes more efficient. In other words, the more activity between the two neurons, the more the connection between them is strengthened. The less frequent the connection the more chance it'll weaken and fall away. Dr Candace Pert says, 'You're literally thinking with your body and the words you say, because sound is vibrating your receptors, which actually affects the neural networks forming in your brain. This ability of the brain to rewire its physical structure is known as neuroplasticity – we can, and are constantly, changing our brain and its wiring.' [16] This is a good thing!

In the movie *What the Bleep do we Know?* scientists and physicists talk about how, at a biochemical level, our bodies become addicted to the neuropeptide (nerve proteins) rush that floods our system each time we experience particular emotions. It's this biochemical addiction that explains why we subconsciously keep creating the same realities for ourselves, even when that's not what we want. 'What's wired together, fires together,' says Dr Joe Dispensa in the movie, talking about how connections have built up so that it only takes one thought to trigger off a well-worn complex chemical pathway. When cells that are continually bombarded with a particular neuropeptide later multiply, they duplicate creating additional receptor sites for the neuropeptide we've become addicted to. Receptors are very specific – for example, opium will bind only to opiate receptors – so when we live in a constant state of guilt about our bodies, about broken diets and discarded exercise programs (and the myriad other things Dietonians feel guilty about), we increase the receptor sites specific to receiving 'guilt molecules'. There's also a corresponding decrease of receptor molecules for positive things like love and nutrition – or a group of receptor sites may become desensitised so that, to satisfy the increased number of sites for that specific neuropeptide, we need progressively more of the neuropeptide to get the same rush. Thus, as Dr. Dispensa points out, we keep choosing people and circumstances that bring these emotions, with their accompanying neuropeptide 'fix', into our lives. We have literally become addicted to whatever our particular human drama is, and in the process our thoughts are literally, changing our biology and forming our bodies via their ongoing chemical messages.

How you adopt your personal cultural standards

So how did your addiction to your particular human drama come about in the first place? Well, let's rewind a bit. At birth your neural pathways weren't formed, but over time, as you collected information about how the world you found yourself in worked, they gradually and strengthened over time.

Of course, what you mainly saw many times over while you were growing up were the repetitive patterns of behaviour that went on in your environment. The more you were exposed to them, the more you became familiar with these conditions, which then become your truth – and the more those neural pathways were strengthened. So, for example, if you were only ever exposed to Chinese writing, your brain would have developed patterns that allowed you to make sense of, and understand, Chinese. But if you later moved to an environment where English writing prevailed, your brain wouldn't be able to make sense of it because it hadn't developed the neural pathways that recognised English patterns. This is how knowledge and cultural standards become wired into our bodies.

So, taking a look at your own environment: was it peaceful and loving activating positive neuropeptides over and over and building neural pathways which reflected your belief that the world was a safe place? Or did you grow up in an angry and hostile environment, so that negative neuropeptides like fear and anxiety became wired into your neural pathways so that you view the world as an unpredictable place?

Those early neural highways became the templates for creating and maintaining our ongoing human dramas because we carry our internal brain patterns with us wherever we go. Even when we come into contact with people having totally different beliefs to the ones we grew up with, we will continue to interpret their actions through our own wired in templates of understanding the world. Thus, if I have been brought up in a hostile world, this experience becomes the filter through which I judge everyone's actions, and even benevolent deeds can be interpreted as malevolent ones. *This is why there really is no such thing as an objective truth; it's all subjective.* The truth doesn't exist in external circumstances; we are all busy creating our own personal truths according to our unique internal neural pathways.

How we maintain our human dramas

Once our brain patterns and corresponding neural pathways have been formed, we go about re-creating our own human dramas by distorting, generalising, taking information out of context or even omitting evidence so that the reality we're receiving is able to match what we already believe to be true. This is what activates our neuropeptide 'fix'.

The average body-concerned Dietonian, whose truth is that no-one could possibly love her, 'hears' people say she's fat when the words haven't even been uttered. She 'sees' people looking at parts of her body she's ashamed of, even when they aren't. She 'imagines' what discussions people are having about her shape or size. She sees someone laughing and immediately 'knows' their laughter is about her body. She walks into a room, a conversation ends and she immediately assumes her weight was being discussed. What she's doing is maintaining and strengthening her personal 'truth'.

Muscle testing for health

Are there tangible ways we can observe and measure the impact of our thoughts and their biochemistry on our health? I believe we can. Kinesiology, the study of muscles and their movement, first received scientific attention through the work of Dr George Goodheart who found that positive physical stimuli (e.g. nutritional supplements) would increase the strength of certain indicator muscles, whereas hostile stimuli (e.g. artificial sweetener) would cause those same muscles to weaken. This implies that the body has wisdom, or a consciousness, way beyond what had previously been recognised – it 'knows' what is good or bad for it. In the 1970s Dr John Diamond's research using kinesiology found that the body even recognised which *emotions* were good or bad for it. When an indicator muscle was tested for a strong or weak reaction, smiling resulted in a strong muscle but when the statement 'I hate you' was uttered, the muscles turned weak.

More recently kinesiology received a further advancement though the work of Dr David Hawkins, author of *Power vs. Force*. [17] His years of research have culminated in a Map of Consciousness – a scale of 'relative truth' according to which almost anything (especially emotions) can be calibrated at specific numerical values between 1 and 1000 using muscle testing. This involves testing the strength of an outstretched, resisting arm by pressing down on it, while making various statements and calibrating the result. When an outstretched arm is tested for strong or weak responses, a kinesiologist can 'ask' the body: 'The emotion anger calibrates at 100 (Y/N)? 120 (Y/N)? 150 (Y/N)?' As soon as the correct calibration for anger is reached, the arm muscle resists the downward pressure being applied to it. (And so on for an entire range of emotions.)

Our body's protection and growth modes

It makes sense that our body would be able to indicate to us what is health-enhancing and what isn't because physiologically, our central nervous system is finely tuned to differentiate between, whether the biochemical messages (neuropeptides) that flood our systems are either supportive of life (busy with growth) or not (busy with protection).

As Dr. Bruce Lipton [18], points out, our cells survival depends on what proportion of the time they spend operating in either 'protection' or in 'growth' modes because his work proves they can't be busy with both functions at the same time. When Dr. Lipton took 2 sets of cell cultures and put them into separate Petrie dishes and then placed either food or toxin in exactly the same position in each Petrie dish, after incubating them, he found that all the cells had changed their biology so as to move either towards the food (=health-enhancing growth) or away from toxins (= health-eroding protection). So while moving away from stress/toxins is a short term survival measure, to stay there for any length of time becomes health-eroding which is why stressful emotions with their toxic neuropeptides impact on our indicator muscles by weakening them.

So long as there is harmony in the community of cells that make up our body, health-enhancing, muscle strengthening, cell growth, maintenance and reproduction are occurring. However, when we're stressed or fearful, our cells react to this 'toxin' and revert to 'protection' mode which automatically shuts down the growth processes. Dr. Lipton points out that we have two protective mechanisms: one protecting us from internal threat (our immune

18

system which protects us from virus and bacteria and fights cancer cells etc…) and one to protect us from external threat (our adrenal system which is activated when we are in a fearful, anxious or perceived stressful situation). Our external protection is controlled by the HPA (Hypothalamus, Pituitary gland and Adrenal system) axis.

For example, you're being chased by an assailant, and are going to need your arms and legs to protect you. Because stress hormones constrict the blood vessels in our gut, your body's energy (nutrients), instead of being utilized in growth are now suddenly being sent preferentially to your arms and legs to help you flee or fight. Stress hormones also cause our immune system to shut down which is why doctors doing organ transplants also give patients immuno-suppressants to shut off the immune system so it does not to reject the new organs.

As Dr. Lipton points out from an external protection point of view, our cells work like a city. Most of the time factories are producing, school are imparting knowledge and society is productive. But, let's say its wartime and an emergency siren goes off, everyone heads for shelter and all production comes to a grinding halt for as long as the perceived threat continues. So long as this doesn't happen too often or the threat doesn't continue for too long – the city is able to keep functioning. But what happens if that city perceives itself to be under constant external threat? How long can supplies last with no new production?

Just like this city, our bodies are designed to spend very limited time in protection mode and the vast majority in growth mode. The emergency siren going off can be catching ourselves in the mirror and feeling fear because: "no-one could possibly ever love this fat body!" Our external emergency siren is triggered by our perceptions which in turn trigger our biochemistry so that the neuropeptides flooding our system send our cells scuttling into protection mode. The Hypothalamus is that part of the Central Nervous System that perceives the environment, allocates a survival value to everything and then decides whether to put our cells into growth or protection mode. When the Hypothalamus perceives a threat or stressor, it alerts the Pituitary gland (the master gland) which co-ordinates the functions of the 50 trillion cells that make up our body by sending a signal to the Adrenal gland to release stress hormones which close down our growth mode. The problem is that in modern times, we spend so much time stressed to the hilt (especially if you're a Dietonian) that we're spending vastly more time in 'protection' mode than we should. Stress increases the wear and tear on our cells and in addition, the longer we stay in 'protection' mode, the less our bodies re able to replace the cells we loose every day.

The value of Dr. Hawkins's Map of Consciousness is that it divides all emotions into either high-energy attractor patterns that release health-enhancing endorphins (these keep us in growth mode), or low-energy attractor patterns that bio chemically release health-eroding adrenaline (these put us into protection mode). Key to the Map's development was the discovery that all negative emotions as well as anything that is fake, artificial or false resulted in tested muscles instantly going weak – at a calibration of 200 or less. Positive emotions, original works, organic products and honesty all calibrate above 200, and result in muscles testing strong. Love calibrates at 500 and peace at 700. The numbers however, increase in a logarithmic rather than an arithmetic way, meaning that even an increase of a few points represents a major difference in power, so love, calibrated at 500, is not measured as a simple 300-point increase over the 200 level.

Dr Hawkins' research gives evidence that when our thoughts produce high-energy attractor patterns (positive attitudes like love, compassion, and acceptance), they lead to muscle strength, a strengthened immune system and vibrant health. On the other hand, thoughts that produce low-energy attractor patterns (negative emotions like resentment, anger, fear, anxiety), weaken muscles, and ultimately result in disease and illness. His work physically illustrates our biological underpinnings, known as psychoneuroimmunology – the study of how emotions, the brain, our cells and neural pathways work as one single unit in order to determine our health (psycho = mind; neuro = nervous system; immunology = immune system).

Secret messages of water

Still focusing on this fact that everything, including thoughts and words, has vibrational frequency that impact on our body in health-enhancing or health-eroding ways, there is also another surprising source besides kinesiology that gives us a peek into what might be occurring in our cells to make them test either weak or strong. *The Secret Messages of Water* chronicles the work of Japanese researcher Dr Masaru Emoto. [18] He photographed the effects that pre-recorded words had on distilled water. When water was exposed to words like 'love' and 'gratitude' (high-energy attractor fields), it formed magnificent strong crystals, yet a phrase like 'you stupid fool!' (a low-energy attractor field) produced only a broken pattern. When water was exposed to a negative television show it also produced disordered crystals whereas a wholesome show once again produced a fully formed crystallised pattern.

Music and the body

Classical music (high-energy attractor) also produces beautiful crystals whereas heavy metal music (low-energy attractor) produces disorganised ones. That certain types of music have a beneficial affect on the body has been well researched. 'Music therapy research has demonstrated beneficial effects on the cardiovascular system, pain perception, stress and endocrine activity. Music therapy has been shown to increase salivary antibodies in hospitalized children after only a single session.' [19] Dr Candace Pert says that music resonates directly with our receptors, setting in motion all kinds of cellular activities so that we are, literally, 'hearing with every receptor on every cell in our bodymind and not just through our ears' ('bodymind' implying both the physical and emotional brain-related aspects fused as 'one body'). [20]

If high-energy attractor words (like love and appreciation) and music creates beautiful crystals in distilled water, imagine what they could do in our cellular water given that the adult body is about 70% fluid? And does the quality of our cellular water not play a vital role in the quality of our health? If strong crystals (formed by high-energy attractor emotions) are health-enhancing, and broken patterns (from low-energy emotions) are weak and harmful to our health, how might various thought patterns impact on our blood pressure and cardiovascular and immune systems? What's happening in our cells when we bombard them with neuropeptides created by hateful and self-critical thoughts? And when we engage in these negative thoughts day in and day out, does this not have a significant impact on our health and mortality rate? Then again, what happens to our health and mortality rate when we continually immerse ourselves in kind, accepting and self-loving thoughts? These are some of the questions I've been asking myself.

So, Dr Candace Pert and the various scientists featured on *What the Bleep do we Know?* give us the physiological explanation for how our emotions govern our bodies. Crystals formed in water give us an intriguing view of how emotions possibly impact on our cells form a strong or a weak cellular structure. Kinesiology shows us the observable impact emotions have on physically weakening or strengthening the body. Our minds create our emotions and our emotions affect our bodies. Thus, *creating, enhancing and maintaining your health starts with your MIND.* This is the totally disregarded aspect in our body battles as thinness via the 'eat less and exercise more' regime has become the unquestioned method towards which our health efforts are geared.

Looking after your immune system

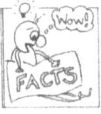

This is not all, though. There's even more proof that our moods impact on our body's chemistry and, ultimately, our immunity to ill health and disease. Studies show that anger and hostility (remember the closed factories as our cells go into survivor mode and the chaotic crystal scenarios?):

- decrease lymphocyte production (white blood cells that help the body fight infection);
- inhibit natural killer cell activity (white blood cells containing enzymes that can kill tumour cells); and
- reduce the antibodies found in our saliva (which is our first line of defence against germs).

The more antibodies we have to fight off germs, the less infection and disease we're likely to fall prey to. In contrast, emotional states such as appreciation (strong crystal patterns) boost immunity – which can be scientifically measured by the quantity of antibodies found in saliva (also known as Salivary IgA) [20]

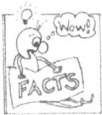

In 1995, the HeartMath Institute in Boulder Creek, California, published the following research. Salivary IgA, heart rate and mood were measured in 30 individuals before and after they experienced 'care' or 'anger', either self-induced (through imagination) or applied externally (via video tapes). To evoke the emotions of caring and compassion, one group was asked to imagine heart-felt appreciation for someone or something, while the other group watched a video of Mother Teresa's work. Both groups responded by producing more antibodies. However the group who *imagined* heart-felt appreciation had 50% more salivary antibodies than those who watched the video (in both groups this was increased substantially when they were exposed to positive music).

This finding reiterates what Dr Emoto and Dr Hawkins have noticed; that positive thoughts and music are high-energy attractor patterns producing magnificent crystals and resulting in strong muscles, all of which determine good health.

The telling factor, though, is that in both the caring and angry groups, it wasn't only the impact of positive versus negative energy patterns that was significant. In *both* groups, the relevant emotions were vastly more powerful when they were *self-created* through imagination compared to those induced externally.

The other interesting finding quoted in this body of research was that ongoing minor mood fluctuations – like those experienced by the average Dietonian going through life in a body she dislikes – are more strongly correlated with disease and illness than are the major stressors. In addition, researchers have found that salivary antibodies reduce in number when there has been a withdrawal of social support. So we might well ask, What happens to our antibodies when we perceive others withdrawing from us because we judge ourselves as unlovable because we are overweight? (Remember that if this is our truth, we'll find evidence to support it and because our brain doesn't know what is real and what is imagined it will send off the same chemical as if it *were* the truth). And what happens when we compound this by not only withdrawing support from ourselves, but also by living with self-induced self-criticism so that our mood is continually spirally downward as we go through life?

In the groups asked to imagine an angry or frustrating incident, the mood disturbance and heart rate were significantly increased, but there was no increase in salivary IgA levels. And they also felt much more anger than the group who watched a war video. In addition, the effect of the anger wasn't limited to when it was being stimulated; the anger suppressed salivary IgA for up to five hours. Where the care and compassion groups reported feelings of love, appreciation and tranquillity, the anger/frustration groups reported accompanying negative physical symptoms, including headaches, indigestion, muscle pains and fatigue, along with their emotional resentments [21]. Think about it, how often haven't you felt angry only to feel a headache coming on, or had an argument at the table only to get indigestion? It's your body is immediately responding biologically with small symptoms of being at dis-ease with itself. When you engage in any low-energy attractor patterns, it's as if your body is jumping up and down, waving a red flag to get your attention, saying 'Hey, stop! You're flooding me with neuropeptides which aren't good for my health. I'm giving you symptoms to warn you of what this could lead to!'

Mind becomes matter

As Dr Pert points out, and the above research supports, it only takes minute biochemical processes cascading through our cellular system and passing on instructions that rearrange our cellular structure, for large changes to occur on a major level. Changes such as antibody-forming, muscle-strengthening crystals or antibody-suppressing, muscle-weakening disordered patterns. Dr Pert takes it even further. She makes a specific claim that raises the whole 'mind over matter/fatter' idea to new levels. To be brutally honest, if this claim had come from anyone other than someone with her rigorous scientific background, I would probably have given it little credence.

Dr Pert states in *Everything you need to know to feel Go(o)d*, '*I actually have come to believe that mind becomes matter.*' Stop for a second to read that sentence once again and take a moment to think about what she really is saying. What we think literally determines our physicality. This is BIG, particularly because Dr Pert is not some woo-woo New Age guru. She is a scientist with over 250 journal publications who has studied the body's biochemistry since the early 1970s.

Remember those Dietonians who said they'd rather give up a year of their life than be fat? Well, ironically, the stress of living constantly in a body you dislike may well mean you're giving up a lot more than a year of your life purely by the eternal worrying over your body. (And here I'm not even taking into account the mortality effects of yo-yo dieting.)

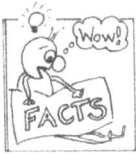

You see stress not only frays your nerves, it also erodes your genetic DNA as well. A 2004 Californian study examined the chromosomes of 58 women, between the ages of 20 and 50, subjected to varying levels of stress. [22] Researchers regularly measured the length of their DNA (telomeres), which shortened with each cell division, thus limiting the number of times a cell can divide (and a person can grow or regenerate). The high-stress group had shorter telomeres compared with the low-stress group, translating into nine to 17 years' worth of ageing! The conclusion? The more stress we are subjected to, the more it impacts on our health, the faster we age and the sooner we die. [22]

Let's take a typical resident of Diet City who, when she was 14, overheard her brother telling his friend: *My sister's bum is so big it looks like the back end of a bus.* Those 15 tiny words are still colouring and controlling her life, harming her health in multiple small ways even though she's now 20 years older.

This Dietonian gets up in the morning, contemplating her need to go for her scheduled medical check-up, where (in her mind) her doctor will see her 'enormous' butt. She 'knows' the doctor is going to judge her, and lecture her to lose weight. Neuropeptides associated with fear and shame trigger her neural pathways, her blood pressure shoots up, her antibodies go down and she feels sick to the stomach. She catches her image in shop windows, notices how her clothes catch on her 'huge' butt and another cascade of shame and self-disgust neuropeptides trigger cellular changes, weakening her muscles and shortening her DNA telomeres. She's in constant stress over when, what and how much she is eating and who is watching and judging her. At the thought of her weekly weigh-in at her slimming club, she feels dread at having her weight statistics read out. She's in a state of hyper vigilance, forever trying to conceal her rear which she perceives to be the target of everyone's stares. The thought of love-making pops into her consciousness, her heart starts beating in her throat. How can she avoid baring all and having hands touch her flesh? Even though her partner denies it, she 'knows' he hates that fleshy rear, so she withdraws from even his best attempts to support her. She gets her neuropeptide fix again and again since her brain is acting as if this is real. This same woman flips through the pages of the latest glossy magazine, notices what beautiful butts all the models have and yearns to have the 'right' body. Her mood plummets with hopelessness as she despairs at ever attaining the perfect 36-24-36; little realizing it's her own internal judge and jury that keep tripping her up. The enemy isn't 'out there' it's 'in here' – it's wired into her belief system. She's creating it. Stimulated by these low-attractor energy patterns, her biochemistry is in overdrive, flooding her system on an ongoing basis with neuropeptides racing from cell to cell through her body.

How might her cells' molecular structure appear? And if tested, how strong her muscles would test? What is happening to the number of antibodies in her saliva and her DNA telomeres? And what is happening to her health?

Keeping on course

Your own internalisation of what you grew up to believe keeps you subconsciously creating, over and over, the circumstances that provide you with your neuropeptide rush. Now, if a pilot flies 1° off course for five minutes, the change might be relatively small; if he continued for five hours, the change would be enormous. In the same way, an occasional negative emotion will have only a minimal impact on the energy flow to your various organs. However, ongoing immersion in low-energy attractor emotions (shame, guilt, anxiety and fear related to living 24/7 in a body you dislike), results in an ever-increasing weakening of your personal power and your immune system. What if this is impacting much more on your health than the actual food you eat, exercise you do or weight you carry?

Granted, escaping the diet superhighway with all its low-energy attractors is supremely challenging in the light of a culture that so highly values progressively smaller and thinner bodies. This comes together with the demand for instant fixes. Any method that doesn't promise instantaneous results we immediately discard as worthless. *What if self-love, kindness and acceptance, tolerance and gentleness towards yourself were the very ingredients that could change your internal chemistry and drastically improve your health and help you escape Diet City?* What if positive emotions *are* the key to survival and health, only your current paradigms are keeping you from considering the possibility? The Joy-Filled Body aims to help you hold these self-loving high-energy attractor patterns of thought over long periods of time – just like that pilot changing course – and often in the face of opposition.

Your thoughts and your health

What is absolutely key to your health is this: *living a life of supportive or non-supportive emotions is motivated not by your external circumstances but by the internal choices and interpretations you make.* The answer is not out there but within. What you conjure up in your mind is powerful stuff and has a profound effect on you. The good news therefore is that the power to enhance your health lies totally within *your control.*

Let's then take another look at that group of rural black South African women. In the 1980s, to be ample in size was considered desirable and beautiful in rural black South Africa. In this culture, fat means 'being healthy, not having AIDS, being fertile, sexy and womanly enough to attract a husband who is wealthy enough to provide well'. [23] In this culture fat women don't live with the ongoing emotional stress of living in a body that is continually insulted, stigmatised, rejected or hated either by themselves or others. As a result, their parasympathetic nervous system doesn't constantly releasing chemicals like adrenaline, noradrenalin and cortisol, which are bad for health. Such chemicals increase heart rate, constrict the arteries and veins, increase blood pressure and suppress the immune system.

Could the lower mortality rate as observed by the Royal College of Physicians amongst these overweight rural South Africans not also be attributed to self-loving attitudes come about because a bigger body is honoured, revered and complimented in their culture? *Since they are immersed in good feelings concerning their big bodies, are they not flooding their systems with life-supporting molecules of emotion, thus creating antibodies and strong cellular crystals which are protecting their health?* If this is so, what implications does this have for Dietonians?

And what about the results of the HAES vs, dieting group results? Sure, over the two-year study period they had increased their exercise (which I have absolutely no doubt contributed to their improved health indicators) but they'd also improved their self-esteem. Now given all the evidence of how powerfully positive emotions improve our health, and I cant' help speculating just what role that contributed to their improved health measures.

Your personal choices

While you may not have had much control over what the initial wiring of your brain was, each of you as an adult has the choice of deciding whether you want to live in a friendly or a hostile environment. This is a vitally important decision, because if you convince yourself you live in a hostile place, you'll forever be biased towards finding reasons to be offended which you'll easily find then use as evidence to reinforce your belief. Our environment always provides us with circumstances that match what we believe, because our perceptions match our truth.

You can stop the ingrained neuropeptide rush by replacing an old thought with a new one. Each single time you do this, the once reinforced neural pathway steadily becomes weaker and an alternative, new pathway starts to build up until the old pathway is no longer automatically triggered as it once was. Eventually the old neural pathway falls into decay and your new reaction becomes the one that is automatically triggered. However, the rewiring of the brain doesn't happen overnight, especially as we all have a tendency to fall back into old habits.

The fact is, we can't escape our bodies, but we *can* choose whether or not to obsess about how 'wrong' they are. And we should be grateful for our emotions because they are the clues to helping us grow, change and free ourselves from our chemical addictions. While each Diet City resident's fears may be unique, if you are an 'I hate myself' Dietonian, your chemical molecules of emotion are harming your health. *The only thing wrong with most women I know is that they're convinced there's something wrong with them. It's terrifying to let go of the many agendas we have for our self-improvement, but the truth is, if we have 87 things that we feel we should be 'improving', and then our primary issue is probably more about self-acceptance than anything else.*

Attractive to whose standards

Here's the thing. Not one of us was born with an idea of how our bodies 'should' look, nor were we born with harsh and fearful attitudes about ourselves. These ideas have become internalised after years of being exposed to strong cultural messages about what is a beautiful/sexy body versus an ugly/unacceptable one. Which is why moving from one cultural 'address' to another can create great ambivalence, as many previously rural black South Africans are now experiencing. One now Westernised ex rural black businesswoman put it this way: *I lost a lot of weight after my pregnancy and that was the first time I had ever been thin. When I'm heavier I feel like an African woman.*

Eating disorders are not found amongst rural Black South Africans. Isn't this something we should be curious about? Only those Black women who have moved to the Westernised environment with its Westernised ideals – they read popular magazines, go to movies and are bombarded with media images of the apparently perfect body – become dissatisfied with the shape they were once happy to have and begin to diet. Since the first reported case in 1983 of a Westernised Black South African woman having an eating disorder, the problem has sky-rocketed as young black women (especially those at a private schools or university) strive to look less like their mothers and more like Western girls. [24]

Our culture has immersed us so deeply in its multiple messages that we aren't even aware of how they influence us to hate ourselves and make us willingly pay any price in the name of body-beautiful. [25] I think it's time to stop the madness and start asking some important questions. *What really stand out are these four words: attractive to whose standards?? I found that when I first started this journey, I was comparing myself to unrealistic thing,s like the airbrushed touched-up slenderellas in the magazines! What helped me was to really look around – go to the Mall, or anyplace where there are a lot of people – and really sit and look at them. How many of them would you say have a 'perfect' body? The reality is that we, as humans, come in ALL shapes and sizes, and that we are ALL beautiful!!*

And it's time we started challenging what we believe to be the Truth: *God does not want you to be like anyone else. There is no X or Y cell that is the same, so why are you comparing yourself to someone else? Don't we just do that all the time? Eish!*

As our rural black South Africans reveal, people from different cultural addresses feel differently about different body sizes. Does this mean their culture is wrong because the Western culture is right? I don't think so. In fact, I personally believe we should be scrambling to acquire some of the beliefs they have about bodies – because *until our beliefs change, we will never free ourselves or our children from eating disorders and being yo-yo Dietonians.*

Chapter 3:
♥
What's eating us?

tories of food and eating criss-cross our lives creating the confusing maze that constitutes Diet City. There are many experiences that feed into your subconscious attitude towards food, eating and your body. The morsels that follow illustrate how we love to eat yet feel guilty when we do; or we hate to eat but feel driven by factors we don't always understand. All the diets we try are about treating the symptom (fat) by trying to control external factors:

broccoli + gym = lose weight.

But it cannot work out because we are not factoring in either our biology or what's 'eating us'. To solve a weight problem we need to look inside, because until we understand what is driving us to eat, no diet is going to get us to Nature's Valley. *This thing (I call it the monster) first visited me when I was 21. I had just gotten out of a very bad relationship where my partner was obsessively jealous and controlling, and once I was 'free' from him, I just started eating and eating. Before that I was normal! I loved to exercise and ate when I was hungry. Over the past 10 years I have gone from skinny to overweight, back to skinny and then back to overweight countless times. My problem is I don't know WHY. I don't have a stressful life, my husband is wonderful although very critical and demanding, and nothing really bad needs to happen in order for me to start bingeing. Why can I not stop when I am that size 34 woman, and like a normal person, just stay there? Why can that taste of feeling amazing never taste better than the next packet of Rolos or Magnum ice-cream?* Because we, as humans, need to create meaning it's not enough to know: 'I am fat'. We also need to know: '*Why* am I fat? Why me? What does it mean? What am I doing wrong?' [26]

The physical condition of being fat is carrying an overabundance of adipose tissue but it's our cultural stories that will try to give us the 'why'. The culture we belong to will say, 'It's because you are weak.' Society is critical of people who are overweight, saying they lack the willpower to just stop eating. There is even the belief that the weakness goes further than overeating; that your personal problems are exacerbated by being fat. *My Mother-in-law truly believes that fat people are intrinsically bad -- even evil. When my husband's brother's marriage broke up, she said that it was because his ex-wife was fat!*

These judgements are so pervasive that they become a self-fulfilling and self-reinforcing prophecy: *'You are fat because you are weak and lacking in willpower.' 'But how do you know I'm weak and lacking in willpower?' 'Because you're fat!'*

Sadly, this is heard by people who are capable of putting themselves through torturous self-deprivation. As one Mind over Fatter group member told us: *'All diets work, if you have discipline.'* She later admitted to having stayed on her diet long enough to lose 103lbs, and then further restricted herself keeping it off for three years. She followed this up with a diet where she ate only powdered meal replacements for nine months, and then lost yet another 80lbs over three months on a diet that severely restricted carbohydrates and included herbal injections. And you want to tell me she has no willpower? No! No! No! What nonsense! This is not a willpower or self-control issue. What has to happen before we 'get' that?

It's the diet gurus who convince us that is we stick to their program, we have willpower (this is apparently good), but if we can't, we're supposedly weak. The irony is that Dietonians often have *way too much* willpower, sticking repeatedly to crazy diets for way too long in their attempts to reach the destination they think will bring them happiness: Thinland. The truth is combating only the symptoms – the fat, the bingeing, the purging – will never bring you peace.

Cultural myths make us believe it's our eating that's the problem. *If I am happy – I eat. If I am sad, angry, confused, bored – I eat. I eat when I change from doing one task to another. I eat when the commercials stop and the TV show starts. Then I eat when the commercials come back on.*

This Dietonian would believe it's her eating that's the problem – it's not. Food is simply the vehicle to cope with some or other sense of inner dis-ease (that is, not being at ease within ourselves) – and we may not even realize we're experiencing this. It's a dis-ease linked to forgetting that we are Sacred and worth loving regardless. Fad diets fail not only because they are unnatural, restrictive and depriving but also because *they ignore what your body or eating might be 'saying' that cannot be communicated verbally.*

If you're reading this book, then it's likely that food is your 'tranquilliser' of choice, even though the way you experience the underlying feeling of lack may vary greatly. But food, as the real source of nourishment, will only satisfy you when it's a physical hunger you're feeding. If you are using it to satisfy non-tangible needs, it will do nothing for you except increase the size of your body. Food cannot grow your soul.

The road to Nature's Valley, as the morsels in this section illustrate, is more complicated and more challenging than achieving thinness. The journey involves looking at your issues around food and your body as a gift. I can hear you ask, 'A gift?'. You've got to be kidding – my issues are a curse!' I'm not kidding, though. It is understanding those issues that will present you with ways back to your Essential Self. Merely changing your body or eating habits won't transform you into a 'whole' human being. I've yet to find a diet that revolves around inner growth! When it comes to liberating yourself from Diet City, it's not thinness that is your liberator – its change and internal growth that will lead the way out. Without that, you are still trapped by your subconscious reasons for being overweight, which keep pulling you back to dieting and Diet City.

Your subconscious reasons for eating offer clues as to where you need to do the *real* work – in your relationships, in yourself. *'The Joy-Filled Body'* helps you access this inner wisdom. If you binge when you're not hungry, it's a sign that you are desperately trying to self-nurture. So long as you ignore this aspect, merely attempting another eating plan (even if there is an exercise plan included) is heading down another cul-de-sac.

Freeing yourself from Diet City requires uncovering and facing the issues that keep you from recognising your own Sacredness. Its noticing negative landmarks that keep cropping up as you walk the byways of your personal history. It's recognising the buttons that keep getting pressed, making you repeat entrenched behaviours towards food, eating and your body.

And don't be surprised when, just as you've uncovered 'The Reason', you discover it isn't a single issue, but multiple issues all working together. It's like going down a country lane only to discover another country lane that leads to yet another one, and so on. The only thing I can tell you with any certainty is that *issues with food and eating are not about food and eating.* They are external manifestations of the emotional and mental concerns you are subconsciously grappling with which at their deepest core are because we've developed amnesia about our Sacredness. Within each of the morsels that follow lies the potential for each of us to get one step closer to rediscovering our Essential Selves, and that will lead us to Nature's Valley.

Abandoned

I had a great childhood, I was loved and protected. When my brother's addiction was at its worst, I felt my parents chose my druggie brother over

31

> *me. My parents were always worrying about him and I felt like screaming: 'What about me?' I guess I felt my parents abandoned me, left me unprotected. Because I felt they could no longer be trusted to protect me, I figured I had to protect and comfort myself. And I guess I turned even more to food.*

It's bad enough to feel abandoned by significant others, but each time you use food as a way of getting away from a situation, you actually abandon yourself. You avoid the door to your Essential Self. Comfort eating takes you down a cul-de-sac to a final destination where you fee even emptier and more emotionally starved.

When you escape Diet City, what becomes important is being there for you and not causing further hurt by piling on extra layers. Self-love means never to abandon you.

Create a ceremony in which you marry yourself and vow never to leave yourself. You can do this quietly on your own, or you can plan the ceremony, buy yourself a ring (or any memento that signifies your self-marriage) and invite friends and family to witness the event.

Acceptance

> *My husband's parents have never considered me good enough for their only son. It's because I'm not the skinny fashion-bunny they think he should have found. They make hurtful remarks. They insist it's a kind of loving teasing, but it doesn't feel that way to me. When they come to visit, I can feel myself eating more. If I'm going to let them into my world, then I'm going to test that they can accept me for the 'me' that I am – the me that is a fat (okay, make that plump) Plain Jane and still eating. I want to be respected for the person I am inside and not the way I look on the outside.*

Just remember: you can only be hurt by the judgement of others if, at some level, you believe at what they're saying. Try treating criticism as a potential gift. Unwrap it and examine it. Take the attitude of: 'Could this possibly be of value to me?' If it is valuable, then keep it and allow it to guide the changes you'd like to make. But be sure this change is a gift to *yourself* and that you are choosing to keep and use it because *you* want to and not because you feel you should. Then it can be priceless.

Your worth should not be determined by the words, actions or reactions of another. If what he or she says or does doesn't resonate with you, then don't absorb it into your being. You don't even have to convince the person that you're not what they think. When we feel offended we're mistakenly allowing another's judgement to be applied to us personally. But this should only happen if we can use it to transform and grow. Self-love is refusing to be offended or take things personally. When we do this, a magical thing happens: those who don't seem to approve of us either change or start to leave our lives.

There's a story about Buddha who, day after day was consistently loving and kind to a fellow traveller who was only derogatory and insulting in return. Finally the traveller asked, 'How is it that you are able to be so loving and kind when all I've done for the past three days is dishonour and offend you?' Buddha replied, 'If someone offers you a gift, and you do not accept it, to whom does the gift belong? When someone offers us the gift of criticism, and we refuse to accept it, that criticism obviously still belongs to the giver. And why would we ever choose to be upset or angry over something that belonged to someone else?'

When we feel good enough about ourselves, our feathers don't become ruffled by what others think about us, and it's like waking up to that quiet centre within, finding a sense of inner peace and contentment, and our need to appease that heart-hunger with food disappears.

Achieving

When stuff is going badly in my life, or even just going so-so my Inner Caretaker is very strong and present I treat myself with kindness and loving care. But when something happens that's good, I suddenly withdraw all my support from myself. Simply put, I treat myself much worse when I encounter success. I become negligent at best and abusive at worse. But I'm just sick and tired of the utter shame and self-directed cruelty I experience when things go well for me. I have just s much of a right to treat myself with joy and kindness when I get a promotion as I do when I have a really bad day.

We both create, and attract to ourselves, whatever situations mirror our internal beliefs, so it's easy to create a life that reflects back to us our belief that we aren't worthy of anything other than bad situations. Living hard is a habitual way of life for Dietonians, who continually expect life's next sideswipe or the next disaster to strike.

There is a famous dual image of a face that, depending on your perception, appears either to be an attractive young woman in a feathered hat or an old hag with a crooked nose. One-half of a room is shown the old hag in the image, and the other half is shown the young woman, then they are pointed towards the duality of the picture. The side of the room that saw the young woman first is still drawn to that image, while the side of the room that first identified the old hag tend only to recognise that image. What they see has been affected by what is already imprinted on their neural wiring. Now think about this in terms of what you see, or you've programmed yourself to see when you look in your mirror– a hag or a beauty?

If you believe that life is hard – that what you're seeing is the old hag – your subconscious is on the alert for the tiniest titbit of information that proves you correct. Your hyper vigilance for evidence will make sure you find it – even if you have to build a mental bridge to make what you find fit what you believe. The more 'evidence' you find, the stronger your belief becomes that life is hard, and then you try to 'eat' it better. If you weren't so hyper vigilant, much of what you pick up on would pass unnoticed; the underlying belief would start losing its grip. You will also have a tendency to overlook information that could change your belief, because you choose from multiple possibilities that which is closest to what you already believe.

Become a detective. Be extra vigilant about information that goes *against* any belief that robs you of happiness. Keep a written record of your findings. This makes them more concrete and less easy to forget. Refuse to put out thoughts that keep you trapped in Diet City. Instead put out to the world the sense that you deserve to live a comfortable and wonder-filled life.

Addiction

You name a diet and I'll bet you I've done it. The scary (sad?) thing is that I am at a totally normal weight and have been for years. But the obsession, bingeing, self-hatred and what I am coming to see as diet addiction have gobbled up the last thirty years of my life.

I believe that we are not addicted to food per se, but the promises of diets – and the belief that maybe this time, we'll get lucky.

Where the drama of food and our bodies consumes us, we are literally addicted to lives of quiet desperation. Self-love is seeing that it's not food and eating that are so problematic to Dietonians; rather it's the fear that you are unlovable unless you diet yourself to a particular level of thinness. When you wrap your hope around diets, you wrap your life around deprivation, restriction, calorie-counting, weigh-ins and constant body worry. These are signs of you feeling you're not achieving enough; you aren't loved enough – that you, personally, are not enough.

Take a long hard look at where, in your life, you are not getting enough, or whether you feel as if you are not good enough.

Ageing

The older I get the more despairing I become about my weight and shape. Just thinking about growing older is enough to send me off on a doughnut-devouring spree. Every birthday marks the marching on of time. . . I'm another year older, with only more wrinkles and the effects of gravity to show for it.

Refuse to buy into the belief that birthdays merely signal a period of decay! When you live in Nature's Valley, anniversaries of your birth are also a reminder of your ability to rejuvenate. Remember the old hag you sometimes think you see in the mirror? Self-love is looking at that same face and seeing something different: wrinkles can be laughter lines as well as a record of your rich and amazing life.

You have a choice as you grow older: to grow more conscious either of age or wisdom. Age is merely physically marking the passing time on a calendar - growing old is marking decay on a mental calendar. You don't stop playing and dreaming because you're old –you grow old when you consciously stop playing and having dreams.

Look on your wrinkles and the effects of gravity through kind eyes. So what if your breasts are having a race to see which one is able to tuck itself into your waistband first? When you're living in Nature's Valley, you'll realize that yours aren't aberrant. Around the world there are other sagging breasts and tummies doing what body bits naturally do. Focus on *preventing* growing dissatisfied and boring, instead of homing in on fears about your ageing body. Be more concerned about losing your dreams and sense of humour than your looks. Laughter and some zaniness will do a lot more to keep you feeling young and vibrant than body worry ever will. Focus less on the cellulite that drives you crazy and more about not living crazily enough. When you are lying on your deathbed, you are likely to think not of the things you did and regret, but rather the things you didn't do – the chances you didn't take, the times you didn't live as if you were fully alive. So . . . revere instead your life's depth and breadth.

Be self-loving and *go backwards* – divide your age by 10. So if you are 42, you can now be 4.2 years young. This gives you permission to throw tantrums, love yourself despite your imperfections, be silly just for the hell of it – wear a tiara for a day, giggle at the things adults aren't supposed to. Give yourself permission to laugh long, loud and often – preferably until you're gasping for air.

Anger

> I hated competing for my husband's attention. I'd call to him and get no answer, then realize he hadn't even heard me – it was like he'd 'become' the blasted TV. I felt like he had a mistress: that blasted sports channel, ready to gobble up his time and rob us of doing things together. I'd get mad with him and go off on an absolute tirade. I'd feel the fury rising and next thing I'd be storming out the room, slamming the door behind me. Then I'd think, 'Stuff you,' and land up heading for the fridge and stuffing me!

Anger is never really pure anger – it's a mask for feeling frustrated, fearful or insecure. Anger comes from feeling our rights have been violated, or our needs aren't being met, or we are compromising what we believe in. We may avoid, deny or repress our anger because we've been conditioned to believe it's bad to be angry. We fear that letting out our anger will either rob us of control or we will be labelled as being over-emotional and hysterical.

It's okay to be angry! Legalizing being angry is a bit like legalizing food - it's simply one of many human emotions we need to normalise. Anger is not the problem; how we express it *can* be. Your feelings don't have to spill over into a retaliatory or angry reaction.

On those occasions when your anger seems out of proportion to what triggered it, has an old and painful button been pushed? If you take the time to examine it through self-loving eyes, anger can be a constructive teacher and healer. It can be the entry to healing old hurts and unresolved issues that are now ready to be worked on or released. It can help you transform because anger has much more power as a catalyst for forward-moving action than does apathy or despair.

How do you express your anger? Is it helpful or harmful? There are many ways to cope with anger, like going for a walk, punching a pillow, writing in a journal, or listening to music, and they'll leave you feeling vastly better than the eating.

Deep and even breathing will also help – just concentrate on your breath: in, out, in, out. Identify what's triggering your angry re-action and allow it to guide you in deciding what is, and what is not, acceptable to you. Staying with your anger without stuffing it down with food can also be valuable because it allows you to see firsthand that you can emerge on the other side feeling more empowered.

Anxiety

When I'm anxious I get butterflies in my tummy. I've often mistaken these to be hunger signals. One evening before an appraisal I was feeling quite anxious about at work, I felt this fluttery feeling in my tummy after supper, which I thought was hunger. But I knew it couldn't be because I had only just eaten. I decided to work on my jigsaw puzzle before eating anything. In so doing, I found a piece of my own puzzle that helped me recognise what was going on and made clear to me that this had definitely not been a physical hunger. When I feel those anxious butterflies now, I remind myself: 'what will be, will be', and that no amount of anxiety – or eating – is going to help the situation in any way'. I'm not saying my anxiety necessarily always goes away, but at least I don't automatically turn to food to stifle it anymore.

The more 'head space' we give to anxiety, the bigger it grows. It becomes like an unwanted squatter, taking up space without paying rent. Anxiety taps into your involuntary nervous system which regulates things like your heartbeat, breathing and digestion. When you're anxious, your sympathetic nervous system mobilises biochemical reactions (for example, it stimulates your adrenal glands to produce adrenaline), which can cause muscle contractions in your chest or throat, the release of excessive stomach acids, inhibited digestion or the liver releasing stored sugar. They will also make your stomach feel like it has butterflies doing hip-hop. When, like Dietonians, you're out of touch with your body, these signals can easily confuse you.

If you attempt to mask feelings of anxiety with food, you're taking a short-cut. It also won't release you from Diet City. The pressure of the moment is forcing you to dishonour your body's real needs. There are always better ways to deal with anxiety – for example, it would be far more self-loving to do some physical activity that will help dissipate the adrenaline. It will help you more to journal about it.

Don't allow the pressures and stress of your life to make you shoot yourself in the foot. The moment you find yourself tensing up, pull your awareness back to your senses to centre yourself. Feel the texture of an object, smell a flower, listen out for birds beyond your immediate environment, or visually zone in on the minute detail of something near you. Simply refuse to say or do anything that doesn't contribute to feeling more peaceful. Dietonians so often create their anxiety by sweating the small (irrelevant) stuff – like fretting about the muffin you've just eaten. Ask yourself if it will be important to you five years from now. If it won't, then send the anxious thought packing.

Approval

> *I'm shaping my actions to get favourable reactions (like doing what I think others want or putting their needs before mine or constantly giving) because that is how I get my sense of being accepted, my sense of self-worth. If others approve of or value me I must be alright . . . right?*
>
> *I've been trying like a maniac to get into a relationship, seeking approval and love from outside sources and frantically trying to disguise all those hateful parts of myself under food or punishing myself by over-exercising. I'm struggling with self-acceptance. I don't seem to have enough love in my own heart for myself.*

One of the problems with seeking approval is that we have fixed ideas about what that approval looks like. If it doesn't slot exactly into our ideas, we easily filter out what *others* might consider as support. This is especially true when we don't approve of ourselves – or our calling card, our bodies. If you've come from a home where you had to jump through hoops to get approval, being immersed in that approval and the momentarily warm glow won't lodge anywhere permanently. It's as if self-approval is the side of Velcro tape that sticks, and other's approval is the non-stick side. If you don't have the self-approval Velcro, acknowledgement by others has nothing to attach to. You could lose the weight and receive oodles of compliments, but not 'hear' them. It's easy instead to believe you are inadequate, not worthy of the love, faith and trust others try to place in you. Self-love in this case is to no longer chase the approval of others but slow down long enough for self-approval to find – and catch up with – you.

Building self-approval has to be done brick by brick, layer upon layer. It's not a one-day job. A great way to start building it is to identify the values and principles you want to live your life by, and then stick to them even in the face of adversity or temptation. Take the time to isolate what you value in various areas of your life e.g. your marriage, your friendships, your career, your spiritual life and so on. Then determine what actions would indicate to you that you were living up to your values.

Birthdays

> *I know birthdays are meant to be a happy time, but leading up to every birthday, I find myself eating voraciously. Recently I went on a workshop where we were asked to draw a childhood birthday that was special to us. It felt uncomfortable to realize I couldn't remember one. What stood out for me*

was that my parents didn't seem to care enough to make my birthday feel as it were anything special. It was always a time when I felt forgotten and neglected. I live alone but as each birthday approaches, it's as if I feel neglect and non-caring have moved into my house as well, and my eating mirrors that. I start eating in such a way that if my body could register a protest, it would say I was being neglectful and non-caring of its wellbeing.

Birthdays are a time to celebrate the fact that, if you hadn't been born you wouldn't have had this life, you wouldn't be bringing your unique contribution to this world – no matter how large or small. And what you bring to this world has little to do with how you look on the outside. Self-love is to remember that no matter what, the Creator felt you were special enough to be on Planet Earth. No-one else has your fingerprints or your DNA, you are unique and special, and no-one can ever take the place you were created to fill. Even if you think your parents didn't seem to notice your specialness, you needn't continue to perpetuate that childhood message.

So you want people to remember your birthday? Remind them. If you want a party, throw one yourself, and make it something extra special. Relish putting more candles on your cake and count each one as a blessing of abundance. Introduce a personal ritual to mark your birthday. Keep a birthday journal. Write in it for each birthday and record what you have to be grateful about in that year. Each birthday brings an opportunity to rebirth fresh ideas about you.

Boredom

Whenever I felt bored, I would shuttle between my fridge and the desk. I hadn't even realized quite how bad it had become until we visited my parents during the summer holidays. Quite often I'd find myself standing in front of the open fridge. I finally made the connection when my youngest daughter (who was itching to go to the beach) came in and said: 'Come on, Granny, I'm bored, can't we go now?' When my mother said, 'Go and get yourself a piece of coconut ice to keep you busy until we're ready to go,' the penny finally dropped. I'd heard the same things many times as a child. Food had become my buffer from boredom.

I often find myself bingeing when I have time on my hands – and in my case, it is usually a case of giving myself PERMISSION to relax! I eat from the guilt of being lazy and taking a break. I grew up in a household where resting was a sign of laziness and of course I just can't relax without feeling that I should be doing something more useful with my time.

We live in a world where we are led to believe that if we aren't constantly busy, we are lazy. 'The devil finds work for idle hands.' It's apparently better to be an over-scheduled Dietonian, rushing around at a breakneck speed than to have time to be still. Being bored or wanting to relax and do nothing are things we should not be feeling guilty about. Relaxation allows time for reflection and contemplation, time to slow down enough to hear the whisperings in our soul. Boredom may be a sign that you are at a crossroads, so it doesn't necessarily mean you should fill your time with finding more to do, because that draws your focus away again. Perhaps you need to leave a job that is boring you, release people who make you yawn, or live more meaningfully instead simply allowing your biological clock to run out. It could also be a cry for you to connect and relate more instead of forever chasing your tail. The cry of boredom is often asking for you to respond by doing nothing, sitting quietly and surrendering to a relaxed state. Boredom isn't a signal to eat, it's a signal to stop and listen.

When you're bored, it's just your soul's way of getting your attention. Relax into that bored space and allow a sense of peace and tranquillity to fill it. With practice, boredom in sufficient quantity can help you surrender into relaxation – something we all seldom get enough of.

Brainwashing

I know I've been brainwashed into believing that how I look on the outside is what counts. In my more logical moments, I know this isn't true, but I can't seem to detach myself from all the conditioning I've had. I know it's crazy, but I still see thinness as symbolic of a sane, recovered me.

These 'Aha!' moments of piercing the cultural rules that keep us trapped are great to have, but sadly insight alone doesn't always lead to Nature's Valley. What you need is a paradigm shift. Why not re-look at all the 'shoulds' you've been fed – how you should look, dress, weigh, eat; where you should live; what kind of a person you should marry – and challenge their validity? Our beliefs are such an integral part of us that we don't know where the beliefs end and the real 'us' begins. Whatever we were told was right and wrong by significant adults usually has become our uncontested beliefs, and ultimately dictates how we feel about ourselves. We have continual (and often obsessive) internal conversations with ourselves as we try to figure out whether we are acceptable according to these internalised beliefs.

I was amazed to read a newspaper article once that claimed we have internal conversations at a rate of 1200 words per minute. That's 72 000 words an hour, 17 280 000 a day, 120 960 000 a week and so on. Whew! So. . . it's 6:50am and your thoughts are involved in an internal conversation as you examine the dust on your windowsill; you wonder if the guy next door has noticed you; whether a deceased aunt would like the picture frame you made even though she'll never get a chance to see it. That leads to you remembering how the boys teased you in class 20 years ago, and so on. . . And you haven't even had your morning shower! Such conversations shape whether you feel deficient or sufficient, lacking in worth or worthwhile. The conversations are governed by your uncontested internal list. This list of the 'right' and 'wrong' ways of living is what keeps you behind the bars of the Diet City prison, because they reinforce your thinking that whatever is wrong is a defect within yourself.

However, for every person who agrees with your belief of 'wrong' and 'right,' there are thousands of others who have a different viewpoint to you. Challenging your brain-washing can be immensely releasing and healing. Wise people know it's valuable to change their mindset, fools don't.

Ask yourself these questions: Who gets to judge that a size 32 is really better than a size 36? Who gets to decide what differentiates a 'good' body from a 'bad' body? Our Creator? Generations before us? A crazy mixed-up culture? And what would happen if you simply decided its no longer self-loving to no longer buy into those beliefs?

Brutality

My boyfriend would scream and shout at me, and slam my head against the wall. Every time this happened, he'd be hugely remorseful and plead with me to forgive him. I'd 'punish him' by bingeing knowing he couldn't say anything because my eating was in response to his brutality. The only problem was that in reality, I was punishing myself by eating my way into a body I hated. One day, I snapped. I don't know where my fear disappeared to but for those few moments, I was so furious that it activated a courageous lion in my heart. I let my anger rescue me. I felt so empowered that I had stood up to him instead of turning to eating.

'Deep within people dwell slumbering powers; powers that would astonish them, that they never dreamed of possessing; forces that would revolutionise their life if aroused and put into action.' (Orison Swett Marden). It takes strength to endure abuse and self-love to stop it. This body is the only one you're going to have in this lifetime and how you look after it will often be the key determining factor in how it looks after you into the future. Don't allow someone's violence to make you brutalise your body still further – because you are treating yourself no better than he or she did. You deserve better. When you grow your love of self, your capacity to tolerate poor treatment will plummet and you'll no longer tolerate poor or abusive treatment.

Change

There were big changes going on. We were emigrating, I had to pack up my home, retrench staff that had been with me for years and say goodbye to all my friends and family. It felt like the foundations I'd built were turning into shifting sand and my eating shifted up a couple of gears. I needed to feel as if I were more solid and more grounded, and the only way I felt I could do this was to grow my body into a more solid form. A friend suggested I make a list in order to prioritise what needed to be done. Then, whenever I felt like eating, I was to take it as a sign that I needed to tackle one thing on my list. This not only distracted me from eating, but also helped me progressively accomplish what needed to be done.

I once saw a row of previously gigantic eucalyptus trees that had been chain-sawed off at stump level at some time. They didn't die – instead they adapted and changed in quite the most glorious way. They sprouted multiple boughs and grew into very different trees than they would have been, with only their stumps holding the memory of their previous life. We, too, can not only survive drastic changes, but also sprout and grow in multiple new ways that could enrich our lives. Change can be a time of exciting adventure.

The only thing constant about life is that it's forever changing – and that applies to our body too. It's impossible to make deep changes and properly fulfil your purpose in this lifetime by remaining an unchanged version of what you are. When you stop changing, you stop growing. However, all of us have great ideas about changing others or changing the world, but when it comes to changing our own circumstances or changing ourselves we're often reluctant. We want to hold onto beliefs that are dear to us, which is why Diet City can feel more comfortable to stay in; we get into our comfort zone. Change brings in fresh blood, new ideas and a chance to alter old habits in a new context that always makes maintaining them easier. It's a sign of strength and trust in the Universe to go along with changes instead of resisting. It's our inclination to resist change that causes an even bigger problem – what we resist persists and often grows. In the end most people change, not because they see a door opening but more because they realize a door has banged closed.

Live according to the belief that change is good, that it is to be welcomed. Remind yourself that the only constant is change, so instead of seeing doors shutting be on the lookout for new doors opening.

Choices

People of colour didn't have much opportunity in South Africa a few decades ago, so it's understandable that my father pushed me to succeed. Most of my life has been about what I should do. I live in a time where young Black women have so many choices, yet I was still feeling like I didn't really have choices in my personal life. The overeating has partly been a rebellion against this. But when I started listening to myself, I realized I have choices. I can choose how to live my life! I can choose what I want to eat or not eat. I can choose to have body fun. I can choose to be fat or thin. I'm not advocating total chaos here. I am fully aware that I will have to accept the consequences of whatever choices I make and I want to make choices that are good for me. I suspect that as I start making more choices I really want to make, I will eat less. I have the choice to be kind to myself and to not abandon my hurt and anger to unconsciousness, numbing myself through a binge.

We can either be 'at choice' (where we choose what we want) or we can be 'at effect' (where others or circumstances choose for us). It self-love to be 'at choice' because then we act proactively, not reactively.

Write 'I can choose' or 'I have choices' on cards and stick them where you can see them. They will remind you that you have, and can, exercise choice.

Co-dependence

I've been seeking validation from men – it's like I'm co-dependent on them to validate my worth. I'll have sex thinking that I'm getting love. But what I really want isn't the physical act but the things that come along with it, the acceptance, approval, love, loyalty, having someone I can take care of (fix?). I tend to view these things as unhealthy because I'm coming from a place where I don't have them myself. Being co-dependent on others makes me a volatile, reactive person who gets hurt easily, turns to food for comfort and then blames them for everything including my eating. I want to be with someone because they enhance me, not because of the need to be supported or made complete. I want to be whole myself.

Our culture, through the images it uses to portray love, sets us up to be co-dependent in our relationships. It's all moonlight and roses with delicious wild sex leading to euphoria. If we aren't feeling this ecstasy, apparently we aren't in love. We need to 'become one' with another; we're encouraged to lose ourselves, not *be* ourselves!

Nonsense! Love isn't about tightening your grip on someone, rather, loosening it. If all the love songs are to be believed, true love lasts forever with no effort. Not so! For relationships to last, they take effort and compromise. It's about being able to respect, honour and maybe even take pleasure in the differences that make us each unique and special. Cultural portrayals of love don't encourage us to accept that we are individual and separate, and that any healthy relationship needs to have boundaries. Feeling as if you cannot live without the other person is not love, it's an addiction. Many of us go through life wasting effort in trying to make the reality fit the myth, only to experience frustration and pain – not because what we have isn't good but because we have unrealistic expectations. *Needing* a partner in order to feel whole isn't good for you.

It's self-loving to love with detachment rather than with attachment. You could question whether it truly can be love if you're detached as this appears that you don't care. Nothing could be further from the truth. Loving someone in a detached way means you care *so much* for the person that you don't rebuff or reject them when they don't do or say everything you'd like them to. In effect, this means that your love isn't conditional upon them acting only in ways that please you.

Competition & Comparison

My partner's family is obsessed with weight and being thin – and my sister-in-law is the same age as me so inevitably it becomes this huge competition – who is prettier, fitter, thinner, more successful. It is draining.

I hate the competition around looking good. I hate going into public bathrooms and seeing how every second woman has to primp her hair, or refresh her make-up. This isn't only about looking good to feel good, this is about competing. This is about having whole industries out there devoted to making us feel insecure.

No sense of competition can exist if you *don't buy into it*. Unfavourable comparisons are the quickest way to undermine your self-love and your sense of worth. It is precisely because of our uniqueness that we are all so special. Someone will always be what our culture defines as prettier, smarter and wearing better clothes. There will always be others who zoom around in the sports car you'd kill to have, who wear more expensive jewels and whose house is bigger. So what? To your Essential Self none of these really count. Materialistic things don't make others better or happier than you. The gorgeous woman with her fake smile may be in an abusive relationship, unable to have children, or lonely and suicidal. Simply because she appears to 'have it all' on the outside doesn't mean she isn't living with hell in her heart.

We've been brainwashed into believing that our looks drive whether we find a partner or not. Well, the fact is, not only the supposedly beautiful find partners. And being in a relationship is absolutely no guarantee that you'll be free of Diet City or be any happier than you were when you weren't in one. If it's self-love you're lacking, once that initial relationship glow wears off, what you're unhappy over will simply differ. Instead of being unhappy that you don't have a partner, you'll be unhappy about what they don't do, all the things you disagree on and all the ways your needs aren't being met.

When you're filled with self-love, you can be happy with or without a partner. Just because no-one has been fortunate enough to realize what a jewel you are doesn't mean you have to think of yourself as less than sparkling.

Control

> *The more rules the diet had, the safer I felt and the more convinced I was that it must be the answer. Ironically, the more stringently I stuck to the rules, the more out of control my life felt because even the slightest deviation from them, in my mind, added up to having done something almost unforgivable.*
>
> *I've often wondered how much of my binge eating was some kind of balancing mechanism. I was so busy being 'in control' in almost every other aspect of my life that the scales were over-weighted on that side. Naturally there simply had to be something to balance it on the other side. That 'something' was being out of control with my eating.*

Whenever your life is controlled by rigid rules or timetables (like it often is in Diet City), know that the problem is you *need* for control, not the means by which you attain it. Ironically though, *the only time you're really in control is when you've given up the need to be in control.* That is quite a thought to get your head around, so I'll say it another way. The only time you'll feel in control is when you are going with the flow of life – and dieting certainly isn't doing that. You don't have control over what happens to you, but you do have control over how you *react*. So, if something stressful happens, you alone can determine how it will impact on your day.

For example, you come down for breakfast and bite into a muffin. Your partner raises an eyebrow and you immediately feel guilty, defensive and prickly. However, this is the point at which you make the choice that will determine how the rest of your day is likely to turn out. You could lash out viciously, and have that one-line comment mushroom into an exceedingly bad diet day.

Or you could make a more self-loving choice. You could thank your partner for his concern, and then choose to continue to enjoy the muffin, or calmly choose to leave it. The difference is that self-loving choices leave you feeling in control.

There's a secret to being in control, though. You've got about a five-second window period in which to decide what choice you're going to make – a helpful or an unhelpful one! It's these five seconds between an event you're not in control of and how you react to it that holds the key. Next time, stop and count to five before reacting, then calmly ask yourself what the most self-loving reaction would be.

Cry for help

I felt anger towards my parents. My anger was because I felt, how could they not hear my cry for help? Why didn't they see that it wasn't about the food, that it was much deeper than that? I know that as an adult I must take responsibility for my own life – but how loud must I scream for help before someone hears me? I feel like I've been crying out for help in vain. No one has heard my cries but me, so I suppose I need to start listening to myself.

Food and eating problems are a subconscious way of communicating with ourselves or others. We don't think, I'm not getting what I want; let me eat as a way of letting them know! It bubbles up instead from a subconscious place and controls our actions and reactions without us even realizing it. Our eating is usually trying to 'say' on our behalf what we feel we're unable to say in other ways.

If your weight or eating could talk – what words would either of them be saying? What emotions might they describe or speak of? What is either one asking for? Which of your needs are not being met and how else could you 'ask' for help?

Demise of others

> *While my friend spent her life passionately fighting for the rights of women, I've spent the majority of my life's energy addictively hating my body, trying to change it, comparing myself and finding myself wanting. Her death shook me up: life was passing me by, but I wasn't living it.*

Year in and year out, every second we receive the gift of life – with every breath in, we are given a fresh chance to live. If you really stop to think about it, isn't this small inhalation of air one of the most incredible gifts? Without it we die. Yet it's the gift we take most for granted. Now, think about it. Our Creator doesn't say, 'Oh, you're fat so, sorry, you can't have as much breath as that 'good-looking' skinny model over there.' Or 'You ate too much today, so only half-breaths for you!' Or 'Naughty, naughty, you didn't go to the gym today, so no more breath for you until you behave better!' Dietonians, however, restrict and deprive *themselves* of the real living that could be going into each breath.

What wake-up call would help you realize just how insignificant and unimportant your issues with food and your body really are in the greater scheme of things?

Depression

> *When I felt depressed, I'd try to eat myself better. The more I ate, the fatter I became, the more I hated myself and the more depressed I felt. It was like being on a hamster wheel. I saw an article which explained why exercise was a great help for depression. At first, just the thought of even putting on my walking shoes instead of walking to the fridge felt like having to overcome the biggest hurdle. But now it's become easier because walking for as little as even 10 minutes definitely lifted my mood, so as long as I could get myself past putting my walking shoes on, the walking itself wasn't the problem. After a while I started walking my dog regularly. Every morning I'd pass another woman walking her Dalmatian pup and we'd greet each other, and over time we started meeting to walk our dogs together. Now she's my walking buddy, we have a great friendship and if I have a 'down' day, I can offload while we're walking and that seems to do the trick much better than any trip to the fridge ever did.*

Regular exercise (or body-play as I like to call it) releases the feel-good endorphin, serotonin, which is a fabulous stress-reducer. When we have sufficient serotonin, we feel optimistic, happy, and content and fulfilled.

Serotonin fuels the limbic system, which rules the emotional centre of the brain and determines how we see the world. Women have bigger limbic systems than men and need more serotonin than they do. They also use it up much faster. However, men's brains store more serotonin and manufacture it faster. When a woman's serotonin levels are low, she feels overwhelmed, worried, anxious, sorrowful, distressed or resentful – all triggers for impostor hungers that hijack her into eating comfort foods such as ice-cream and pasta, not only because they are usually on the 'illegal' list but because they do temporarily boost serotonin.

However, there are more self-loving actions that would have replenished those serotonin levels without all the extra calories and guilt: talking about and sharing the problem with a friend, doing anything that involves co-operation or collaboration, holding hands or having a cuddle. These are the best ways for women to manufacture serotonin. Activity is a fabulous antidote for stress and depression and it's great for speeding up your metabolism. Walking and talking have multiple other benefits too.

Make a fridge list of everything (music, books, a bath, wearing a particular colour or outfit, an activity) and anybody you can think of that could lift your spirits. Do that NOW. Next time you're feeling down, go to your list and choose one thing from it instead of eating.

Drama

I'm a bit of a drama-queen and the drama surrounding food and my body made my life more colourful. Everyone was constantly giving advice, bringing me new diets, and the latest diet products. It gave me a point of connection with others and their attention made me feel cared for and special. But it also kept me trapped in a large body. Subconsciously, I couldn't afford to get, and stay, thin because I 'needed' all the excitement and drama that went with my stuffing and starving. I would go on diet and lose weight and there would be compliments and attention which I revelled in, but as soon as those started wearing off, I'd find myself going on an eating spree, making sure everyone knew about the latest developments.

My sister challenged me to find something else to talk to her about as she was bored to tears with my diet roller coaster. It forced me to make changes, one of which was joining a belly-dancing class which provided me with all the drama of wonderful costumes, colour, excitement and a connection with others as well as a different topic to talk about instead of my body, dieting, weight and eating.

Most Dietonians never recognise how the drama around dieting become bars holding us in Diet City prison.

Create colour and excitement in other ways: fix delicious, colourful or exotic food and set a beautiful table. Do your hair and dress in ways that inspire you – even when you're not going out or expecting to see anybody. Any actress can tell you how that helps transport them to a magical space – it's a way of performing without all the sideline dramatics of food and eating. If being on stage would bring drama and interest into your life, join an amateur dramatics or theatre group, or a toastmasters or debating group. That way you'll fill your need for drama and excitement instead of it going via your throat and becoming the ample costume that clothes your frame.

Effort

My dietician kept on at me about changing my cooking methods. But it just all seemed so much effort even though I knew that in the long term it would really be good for me. Then I fell down the stairs and a friend came to help me for two weeks. She'd disappear into the kitchen for 20–30 minutes and come back with food that looked, smelled and tasted delicious. She'd lightly steam her veggies – they were yummy. Instead of making rich sauces for her pasta she'd drizzle it with olive oil and balsamic vinegar – it was awesome. By the time she'd left, I felt so inspired that I signed up for a cooking course and loved it. Peeling vegetables feels almost therapeutic and I no longer think of cooking as effortful – it's a way to unwind and relax after work. And eating better gives me much more energy than I had before.

For many of us the journey is three steps forward, two steps back, and sometimes even three steps forward, four steps back. There's a Chinese proverb that says: It doesn't matter if you're moving slowly, what matters is not standing still. So... keep on moving!

It's always easiest to do nothing, but what's least effortful isn't always what's self-loving. It is easy to want the best outcome but *hoping* for it isn't sufficient; it takes sustained effort. Eating that slice of cake because it looks good right now, or not playing because it's too much effort are short-term pleasures that bring long-term pain. To get to Nature's Valley, you need to tap into the wisdom you were born with on eating and being active, that is, going from effortful to fun. Do things that were dreaded previously with a sense of delight.

Think of your body as the house of your Essential Self. How would you feel if the builder of the home you were planning to live in for the rest of your life used poor materials and careless workmanship? Look at yourself as being constantly 'under construction', your own DIY project. When it comes to returning to Nature's Valley, it's the extremely small changes you nail down over time that produce the profound changes.

With each tiny crossroads of choices you're faced with (Should I dash up the stairs giggling like a child or should I take the elevator?), think not about what will take the least effort but which of the choices could bring more childlike wonder and delight into your life.

Emptiness

Four children kept me on my toes, but when the last one left home my life felt purposeless. I felt old and wasted and ate as if I was patching a wound on the inside with a food-plaster from the outside. As I got fatter, I withdrew from other activities as well, until I was even more isolated and even emptier. A friendly do-gooder dragged me off to help our local night shelter. I enjoyed the sense of 'family' I found there. Since then I've joined a book club, play bridge and work in the shelter. It feels like my life is full again.

Find fulfilment in your life rather than fullness in your stomach. If you're feeling empty and that life has no meaning, it's a signal to uncover your dreams. Find out what gives you enjoyment.

Start a journal; make it colourful and fun. Paste in pictures of things you like, or things that remind you of a way you'd like to feel. Decorating your pages with stars and sparkles is a great way to give your inner child the chance to come out and play. It invites inspiration into those empty-feeling spaces.

Escaping

When I think back n the binges I had when I was way younger, it was as if I was in 'unconscious mode'. Maybe it was staying with my parents, being around them arguing, watching my father's obsession with how everything had to be done in a certain way, the controlling environment. My self-image at that stage was less than zero... Maybe that led to wanting to disappear, get away from all that was happening around me, just stuffing my face with whatever I could find.

I was in a gym for the better part of four to five hours a day. You may be thinking, that sounds so robotic! YES, it was, but it was really great for me at the time because it gave me no time to deal with my divorce.

My mom used to joke that the poorest man is not the man without money, but the man without a dream. That made me very rich because I am full of dreams. Yes, I'm a dreamer. And I guess food is part of my escaping reality. As a 15-year-old I wrote a poem about dreaming versus reality, and if I were to paraphrase the poem I'd say: 'Reality is way too harsh so I'll go on eating.'

Focusing on body beautiful or diets and food can all be ways of trying to escape more painful realities. You might say you've always been told: 'Stop dreaming, stop escaping into your imagination.' But escaping reality can be a really important first step to accomplishing a dream. In the words of Muhammad Ali: 'Champions aren't made in gyms. They are made from something they have deep inside them – a desire, a dream, and a vision.' Those great achievers who have gone down in history all had to 'escape reality' in order to dream up new ideas that hadn't yet existed and have since revolutionised the world. So, escape into dreaming about a more wholesome future instead. Dreaming is your mental blueprint and it can be achieved. When you step in the direction of your true desires, the Universe steps out to meet you and help make them happen. For you to escape the hard realities of Diet City you have to dream of a different life, one without scales, lists of legal and illegal foods, deprivation and restriction.

When you need to escape reality, curl up in a comfy spot and allow your mind to take flight into fanciful imagination. Don't edit the possibilities and think, 'This isn't possible.' For those moments become that child for whom anything is do-able with no restrictions.

Failure (feelings of...)

I do something good and I think, 'So what'? What about ALL the other bad things? There are so many more failures than achievements. Recently I got an A for my studies. But I thought, it's a low A, not a high A. I'm striving for 100%, so less than 100% is never good enough, and I sweep my successes under the rug. I feel compelled to eat when I don't do well in exams and tests. It's almost as though I'm stuffing my failure down my throat. I got to a point where I simply couldn't do that to myself anymore. I've decided that any failure is merely a learning experience, a time to take a step back and work out where I can learn from my mistakes.

Would you stop turning to food if you had a more flexible definition of 'intelligence' and 'success'? Think about it this way: We have been schooled to believe that intellectual achievement is a measure of how unintelligent or how clever we are. In our Western materialist culture, intelligence is highly valued in terms of how far you are able to progress in life: how far up the status ladder you will climb, how much money you will earn, how many possessions you will own and how much power you will wield. You are measured by how well you can read, write and compute. Hmm. Surely the true measure of intelligent living lies not in how much you have but in how much joy you pack into your life? Let's make joy and happiness our new measures of intelligence. There is absolutely no guarantee that the great scholastic students will live happy and fulfilled lives. I've had many highly intelligent Dietonians walk into my therapy room looking the picture of unhappiness. I've also worked with children who have low intellectual abilities but who know how be joyful. Having all the material benefits that intellectual success theoretically brings without the joy and spontaneous laughter is as good as having nothing. Self-love is focusing on intelligent living that embraces joy rather than appearance, achievements or material success. No that's a way to leave Diet City.

Feeling a failure? Ask yourself how you could define the situation differently so as to live a life that is more authentically intelligent and joyful – not matched against Western cultural standards.

Fatigue

I'd get home exhausted and convince myself I needed energy. This source of energy just happened to reside in the cookie jar! Then someone pointed out that a lack of water can cause fatigue, and that exercise or a nap could be energizers too. Now instead of eating, I have a mug of tea, just sit quietly in my garden and listen to the birds while I unwind, play with my grand-daughter, go for a short walk with my dog and sometimes I even take a 15-minute power nap. My other energy-drainer was my clutter – magazines lying everywhere, bits of paper and mail on every surface. After I had reorganised this, I felt light and invigorated.

I'm realizing that if you're tired and you don't rest, your body will demand energy to keep you awake, and your mind will want some sort of reward as well, so it won't be enough to eat an apple for energy – you'll probably want chocolate or cake or toasted cheese... I need to take better care of myself. If my body is screaming for sleep, then I need to sleep instead of pressing on.

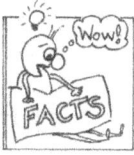

Next, holding onto clutter is indicative of an attitude of scarcity, believing you have to hold onto things in case there isn't enough. Try to adopt an attitude of abundance.

Get rid of energy drainers. Take a page, divide it into two. On one side list everything that is an energy raiser for you; on the other, list all your energy drainers. If you do more things on the energy-raising side, and fewer on the energy draining side, you'll have loads more energy. Clear your clutter. Get rid of the paper you shift around, the piles of opened and unopened envelopes, pens that never write. If you haven't looked at, used or worn items for a year, be ruthless. Get rid of them and you'll find new energy flowing towards you. Set a timer and see how much clutter you can clear in 15 minutes. You'll be amazed at how energising this is. Break down paralysing tasks into bite-size morsels. You'll free up stuck energy.

Fear

I ate and dieted to shift attention away from the real issues. In fact, that's why I eat, to soothe the scared part of myself. But by doing what makes me afraid, I grow. What I realized is that the things I'm afraid of feeling aren't as bad as I thought they'd be; it's the 'not knowing' that's really scary.

Fear happens when we allow ourselves to live in the past or the future. Most of us know the acronym for FEAR: False Expectation Appearing Real. That's true, but I prefer thinking of it as **F**anciful and **E**rroneous **A**nticipatory **R**eactions. You're giving your fanciful negative fantasies so much airspace that your body reacts to an erroneous signal, producing neuropeptides as if you were actually experiencing what you fear.

53

Fear is just a signal that you're recycling past experiences or creating future ones. One of the most powerful liberators from fear is living in the now, where fear doesn't exist. The majority of our fears aren't real, they are created in our imagination, triggering our body chemistry and keeping them alive. Franklin Roosevelt summed it up well: 'There is nothing to fear but fear itself.' But we're so fearful of that early morning weigh-in; we miss the glory of the sunrise or the smell of freshly cut grass. We're so fearful of others witnessing our eating; we don't notice the flavors, smells and textures of our food.

When you're stuck in Diet City, fear is in the driver's seat and you're allowing the right to live life your way to be taken from you. Instead of you calling the shots, fear is. Have you noticed that spending time with fear never reduces those fears; it only makes them bigger. And by not entertaining fear, you're not being fearless; rather, you're deciding that something else has a higher priority. You're not letting fear shut down your choices.

Treat 'The Fear' as if it has a personality that is outside of you. Ask it questions to reveal its tactics, like: Why do you keep bugging me? What makes you grow? What shrinks you? How do you trip me up and trick me into believing you? What and who do you use as your allies? (When you're trapped in Diet City, some of the things you most commonly find are: calories, scales, clothes labels, etc.) What are your enemies? (These could be, say, therapy or no longer comparing yourself with others.)

Put this saying where you can see it often: 'Fear is that little darkroom where negatives are developed (Anon).' Talk back to it, find out what it's up to and don't let its voice get too loud. Then watch for the times when Fear's voice, instead of being loud and insistent, is becoming softer; sometimes it's toned down to a whisper. What has contributed to that happening?

Feelings

I eat when I'm excited, angry, afraid, overwhelmed, sad – all the emotions that I don't seem to allow my body to feel. Today I had crystal healing done, which helped me connect with different feelings in the different energy centres of my body. I felt so released and spacious – but when I got home it was as if the walls caved in and I binged. It feels like each time I get closer to feelings, it's followed by an equal and opposite shutdown and another binge. It feels totally overwhelming to allow feelings to exist because it seems like I'm getting too close to the waves of pain buried inside my body. I guess I am scared of the possibilities of what might happen if I did begin to feel; it's easier to remain closed up!

Often I stuff myself with food or go online and shop so that I can numb my emotional pain away. But this time I decided to let myself feel the emotions instead of pushing them away. This weekend has been awful in some ways, because I experienced a lot of negative emotions. But I said 'no' to that avoidance impulse and 'yes' to looking after myself.

Living in cyberspace and eating sugar has become a way of escaping into another world. I don't know what it is that I want to blot out so badly but I wish I could just leave. I wish dying could be like walking out of a door and just closing it behind you.

A while ago, I was walking along a beach, my emotions as tumultuous as the giant waves crashing onto the shore. I found myself drawn to the actions of the periwinkles. As the powerful waves dragged backwards to rejoin the sea, they pulled with them everything but the periwinkles. These tiny sea creatures use clever tactics to withstand the wave's forces. They don't resist the pull but first roll *with* it until the power of the pull has diminished. Only then do they wave around their 'aprons,' positioning themselves to lie across the flow of the water. Finally they flip over, anchoring their aprons into the sand. Such wisdom!

Instead of trying to resist my feelings, it was more helpful to initially go *with* the flow of those emotions. When I stopped my desperate attempts to suppress them and allowed them to submerge me, I was amazed at how quickly their power started to ebb. By trying so desperately to stop them, I'd only given my negative emotions more power and made myself more vulnerable to being swept away by them. When I put myself in a position to remember the impermanence of emotions (these too will pass), it then became easier to do 'anchoring' work to stop myself from being swept into the negative abyss.

Every time you avoid feelings by pushing them down with food, you do three things. You rob yourself of the ability to prove to yourself that you don't lose control or break down or scream and shout. You simply strengthen your habit of avoidance: feelings = eat. You miss out on the message your feelings are giving you.

Numbing out with food is a Diet City trap. Becoming an observer of the internal chatter that's creating your emotions can change how you experience those feelings; eventually the chatter becomes quiet and a sense of peace replaces them.

To become an observer of your feelings, ask yourself a few questions. If you had to step outside of your body and observe your raging emotion, what parts of the body would you feel it raging in? Can you tell if it has colour(s), shape(s), temperature(s) or texture(s)? In your mind's eye, paint, draw or scribble how it might look if you were an artist capturing it on paper. If you had to step back enough to see the words of the internal chatter that created these feelings displayed on a series of banners, how might this detached observing change those emotions? Alternatively, if you repeat the words to yourself as an observer: 'Hmm, I see I'm thinking that....', how does that change the impact they have on you?

Frustration

> *At the smallest amount of frustration or irritation, I'd head for the bread bin; I could eat eight slices in one sitting! One morning, driving my son to school I got so annoyed with an old man driving too slowly that I almost caused an accident. My ranting terrified my son so much that when we stopped at a traffic light, he got out of the car and refused to get back in again. I realized just how out of control I was and signed up for a stress management course, where I learnt how to raise my frustration tolerance level and take back my power. The key for me was this: the problem wasn't with what was, or wasn't, going the way I wanted it to. It was that I was blowing small things into big things and then reacting in unhelpful ways.*

Unless you are using substances that reduce your capabilities of self-control or you've allowed yourself to get into such a depleted place emotionally, no-one can *force* you to feel anything, including frustration, without your permission. It doesn't get you anywhere to say, '*You* hurt me', or '*You* made me angry.' No-one forced me to be angry or to eat – they are choices I make. If I am hurt, this emotion is the consequence of how I've chosen to interpret the situation. It doesn't help you to make mountains out of molehills because then even the small things immobilize you. When we lose sight of the bigger picture, we compound the problem, living our lives as if they were one big emergency. Be aware of how you give away the power to choose how you feel and how you live your life. Resolve not to give it away to the circumstances and people who most frustrate you. You have the power *not* to do that!

You may not be able to control what people around you do, but you do have the power to interpret people's actions in the the kindest possible way. Try to believe that they're not purposefully setting out to frustrate or irritate you.

When you make kind choices, you're activating strong muscular processes and also health-promoting antibodies. Ask yourself: What interpretation could I choose that would be most healthy for *me*?

Gender roles

I've always been a bit of a midge. I'm short and weighed in at about 95lbs. My weight problems began when I qualified as an accountant and went to work in a very a male-dominated company. It was really frustrating feeling like my opinions had no sway whatsoever, especially when I'd qualified cum laude. Getting larger became my unconscious attempt at trying to have fewer feminine curves and to be a bigger presence so that the company directors would treat my opinions as if they had substance. All I achieved with increasing my body size was shrinking my confidence. So I became a weak-willed fat blonde 'slob' who was still treated as brain-dead. I resigned and started my own business.

Traditionally, women have been taught that their bodies are a powerful bargaining tool. Not so for men: their power comes from status, position and possessions. We can change that! Where we need to add weight is to our personalities – our sparkling wit and wicked sense of humour. If you're in a situation where you feel you aren't respected the way you'd like to be, analyse the situation with fresh eyes.

Self-love is respecting yourself and your own judgement enough to leave if staying is going to erode your confidence. There's no shame in protecting yourself.

In the words of Winston Churchill: 'Attitude is a little thing that makes a big difference.' Do what's necessary to protect your heart, your spirit and your wisdom. Remodelling your body to fit a situation is a temporary fix at best and often only gets you more trapped into Diet-City thinking. Most often, it's not your body that needs reshaping but your internalised beliefs that having a bigger/smaller body is the only way to make a difference (in the long term) to your life.

What parts of your personality would you like to expand? Ask yourself: How would I talk if I was sparkly and witty? How would my voice sound? What look would people see in my eyes? How would I hold my body, my shoulders, and my arms? What would people notice about my mouth and jaw? What sorts of thoughts would I be having? In what positive ways would people be responding to me? How would I be feeling during these exchanges? Paint a clear mental picture for you to model yourself on.

Giving too much

Most women don't take the breaks they need. We feel we aren't entitled to it, or that there's no time, or that the world will collapse if we take time out. Then we stuff our faces with food as a short-term measure against the hunger, anger, loneliness and fatigue. We continue giving, giving, giving. But how can we keep on giving when we're running on empty? Meanwhile, the resentment keeps rising and that resentment shows on the scale or in the size of our clothes.

'Me-time' has been a big issue for me. Even though certain me-times had been agreed on, I always felt guilty about taking them, and I ate to try and numb the guilt. What inevitably happened is that I got sick; then I didn't feel so guilty taking me-time because I had a valid excuse! But was it my family frowning on my 'me-time' – or was it actually me? It was me, desperately trying to be the person I felt I 'should' be: the perfect wife and mother, the perfect worker, and so on. Only now I realize that that person does NOT exist!

Women are generally great givers and poor receivers. We have been culturally infused with values of caring and being there for others, often to our own detriment. We're also often reluctant to ask for help and support for ourselves. Yet to ask for help allows others to know we have a need. It paves the way for us to have that need filled, allowing us to experience the positive emotions of appreciation and gratitude (creating a positive energy flow and stimulating strong muscles). When we are filled with gratitude, we don't need to fill ourselves with food. It also gives the people who care for us the pleasure of sharing and supporting.

It's *not* selfish to put yourself first in self-care. In 2005, I went away for a few days to be alone, armed with crayons, cloth and fabric paint, inner child cards, books that feed me, music that stirs my soul and walking shoes. I had no access to phones or e-mail. My few days delivered way more than I'd ever hoped for. As ideas and thoughts popped up, they found their way onto my cloth in a colourful and unsystematic way. I took long baths and naps any time I felt like it. Sometimes I sat and focused on my breath, feeling grateful for it. I walked and picked daisies to put in my hair or to scatter on my table. I prepared my food with extra love and care. I ate slowly and mindfully, by candle- or firelight, or sitting on the porch with the sun to warm me. The few days passed in a whirl, but I felt like I'd been away forever and had travelled great distances – all the way back to my inner centre. I came away feeling calm, invigorated and deeply in tune with myself. I felt so filled that I had more to give, and there were numerous pay-offs for those around me.

HALT is a great acronym for feeling Hungry, Angry, Lonely or Tired. Stop and take a break – but I don't mean an eating break! Consider this: if you do too much for others, you sometimes prevent them from growing themselves. With the best intentions in the world, you may be disempowering them. Certainly, things may not get done your way, but perhaps there are also other ways to do it.

Ask yourself: if I were to be knocked down accidentally today and landed up in hospital for months on end, in what ways might the people I'm continually doing things for be able to grow?

Take some time out for yourself. If this is impossible, try the follow instead. Take the occasional 60 seconds to HALT, sit quietly and focus on being there for yourself, even if it's just for a minute at a time.

Guilt

When my son committed suicide, the guilt was all-consuming. The more it ate at me, the more I ate. Being a greedy-guts also gave me something to focus on rather than the suicide – something else to punish myself about rather than just the suicide. The guilt at bingeing replaced the guilt of not being good enough as a mother. I wasn't really a horrible mom; I just did what I thought was best given my resources and knowledge at the time. Now, when guilt tries to overpower me, I weed the garden – I am weeding guilt out of my mind. Over the years, my garden has become a place of peaceful contemplation and the place where I choose to honour my son's life rather than focusing on his death.

My brother died of AIDS and I wasn't there for him; the doctors didn't tell me. The guilt ate away at me and food became the Velcro of my life. My life felt like a sandwich, two dry pieces on either side with food as the Velcro in the middle, sticking the two sides together. It kept me from coming apart.

I have always felt awe in the presence of majestic trees. I love that their stories are stored in the concentric rings we see when they're cut through horizontally. These rings tell us which years were drought years and which weren't. If we could see a horizontal section through the body of a Dietonian, I'm quite sure we'd see a wound wrapped within a ring of abundant eating, followed by a ring of guilt, then a ring of restrictive dieting, followed by catch-up eating, and so on. Dietonians have so many things to feel guilty about!

But, in being guilt-stricken, you're wasting a life not bettering it. If I think back about all the things I've felt guilty about, I could pass for a mass-murderer instead of someone simply struggling to have an unrealistic body! Much of a Dietonian's guilt comes about through buying into superficial manmade truths about 'goodness' and 'beauty', but guilt is a wasted emotion if it doesn't change the action – like apologising, turning the page and moving on. Guilt is a major reason for Dietonians not making it to Nature's Valley.

Guilt arises from struggling to forgive you. The fact is, the more self-forgiving you are, the easier you will find it to forgive others. Stop atoning for what you consider to be 'sins' with feelings of guilt. Focus rather on creating personal joy and being of service to those around you. Practise random acts of anonymous kindness – that's way better than wallowing in guilt.

Habits

I first chose my habits. Once they were firmly entrenched, they took over and chose for me. When I got divorced, I'd come home from work, switch on the TV and head for the chips. When a new boyfriend came along, the loneliness was a thing of the past, but the chips and the TV weren't. Changing the position of the TV so it was no longer in my path removed the automatic impulse to punch the TV 'on' button as I walked past; a reluctance to eat on my new couch helped me not to eat in front of TV.

I'm so impatient with myself! I want to be perfect today, NOW! I know it's taken me years and years to form the habits and attitudes I have about food and my body, so I'm struggling with having to take the same, or even more, time to reverse them.

Diets pretend that conquering the weight problem is simple! What the diet gurus don't share with you are the oodles of patience, perseverance and the time it takes to first make the *mind* (neural) changes. Beliefs are entrenched and often unquestioned habits of thought and action. Changing these ingrained habits takes time, especially in our 'instant fix' world. It's too easy to give up, thinking we're hopeless the minute we stumble back into an old pattern. But in her fabulous book - Succulent Wild Women, SARK shares some wisdom from Portia Nelson that I think illustrates most profoundly what the path of change looks like.

So often we're tempted to think it's a linear event. We discover an old unhelpful pattern, we resolve to change it and viola, miraculously it changes effortlessly overnight. This is more realistic.

1. I walk down a street, fall into a hole I didn't see and struggle endlessly to get out, but I'm not to blame.
2. I walk down the same street, fall into the same hole I overlooked and struggle for a while to get out. I'm still not to blame.
3. I walk down the same street, see the hole which I still fall into. I get out right away, I take responsibility.
4. I walk down the street, see the hole and walk around it.
5. I choose another street. And I'd like to add:
6. I consciously choose to walk down the new street over and over.
7. Now I choose the new street out of habit.

This story shows how at first the habits keeping us in Diet City are unconscious (well-established neural pathways), and how, through repeatedly falling into an old pattern with awareness, we can make changes (we start to slowly break down the established neural pathway and 'rewire' a new one). It illustrates that a changing habit is seldom a one-step-wonder but rather a series of repeated stumblings in which we strive to catch ourselves progressively earlier each time. When we finally choose a new street, we establish a very weak, new neural pathway that has to be strengthened. This strengthening is the most important step because old habits easily return – as learning new behaviours doesn't automatically extinguish the old ones. The new behaviour has simply been added to our repertoire.

The old behaviours, despite their weakened neural pathways, are sneakily lying in wait, ready to pop out at us especially if the context hasn't changed. How we act depends on which memory we retrieve. New memories are easier to retrieve than when all the old things that once triggered the actions we want to change are all still around us.

Chapters 6 and 7 deal with the need to practise new behaviours over and over, to strengthen the new neural pathways, until they eventually become the new unconscious habit that's exercised automatically and with ease. Along the way there will be those times when you fall back into the hole; it's a part of the process and you need to keep at it, believing you'll get there.

Herein lies the problem, though. In an attempt to leave Diet City, you have tried so many plans so many times, never realizing you're persisting with the very methods guaranteed to keep you there. Only fatter this time, more psychologically bruised and with less self-belief. Without self-belief, you won't have the patience or perseverance to stick with anything.

Stop believing in diets and start believing in your ability to achieve what you ardently want, and then enthusiastically act on it. Apply a lack of persistence to dieting – that's an absolute prerequisite for escaping Diet City!

> *Everyone talks about how they comfort eat. Not me! I ate when I was happy. Growing up, family celebrations always revolved around what we ate. Some of my happiest memories are of us sitting around our huge table. It never occurred to me that there could be alternative ways to celebrate until we had a treasure hunt for Easter – I loved the activities. Now when I plan a celebration, I first plan what we are going to DO, and the eating takes secondary place. Food is absolutely always a part of it, but the focus has changed from 'What are we going to eat?' to 'What are we going to do?'*

Just because, according to tradition, celebrations have always revolved around food, it doesn't mean that's the way it has to stay. You can change the focus, as this Mind over Fatter pilgrim did, and celebrate in inventive and interesting ways whilst still maintaining all the ingredients that make get-togethers and celebrations wonderful: connecting, laughing and memory-making. Get your children involved in helping you come up with fun ideas for your next family celebration – they'll love to feel a part of it.

One of the most fun evenings I had took place when I was about 12. We cleared the chairs from around the table and played a ping-pong game where you'd hit a ball across the table and pass the bat to the next person and run around the table to the other side. Each time anyone missed their ball, my mother progressively spelt wrote the letters D-O-N-K-E-Y onto our cheeks, arms and faces in lipstick. Once anyone had all the letters for 'donkey', he or she fell out of the game so that it became progressively more difficult to hit your ball and get around to the other side of the table for your next ball. Everyone, including the adults, screeched with laughter. We made wonderful memories we'll cherish forever that night just by being a little crazy.

Practise what Swami Beyondanda, in *Duck Soup for the Soul*, calls 'FUNdamentalism'. This is about placing a lot more emphasis on the FUN than the mental. If you have any people in your family who were weaned on a pickle, encourage them to lighten up and take themselves less seriously. One of the biggest reasons Dietonians are unable to free themselves from Diet City is because they take the whole issue of their weight way too c-4-ceriously (okay, seriously). Just get in touch with that fun-loving six-year-old inside you, dying to get out. Be much more serious about playing and play less at being serious!

Make your celebrations an adventure rather than just an eating spree - play fun games. Take turns at inventing daft new words for others to make outrageous guesses as to their 'daffy-nitions'. For example: a 'sqircle' could be a square circle; others might say it's a squid with an ircle (whatever that is). It's not about necessarily guessing the right answers nor is there an object to the game except to laugh and have FUN! If there's a bookshelf in the room, have one person start a story using the first title. When they stop, the next person has to continue with the story however they choose, but it has to include the title of the adjoining book, and so it continues until you've gone through all the book titles. (And for those pickles who think games are silly – they're also good for mental agility.)

There are old-fashioned games like 'pin the tail on the donkey' or 'hopscotch'. Give each person a streamer to throw at one another while yelling out something they love or admire about the other person, creating a fun spider's web of colourful connection. And, yes, it will be noisy and unruly!

Holey heart

I have consistently driven men away with my super-neediness. I used to be super-high maintenance; now I'm just high maintenance. Ha! Ha! When I'm in a romantic relationship, I don't comfort eat quite as much, because I'm getting lots of hugs and physical affection. I have this big need for hugs, and when I don't get them on a regular basis, I eat and eat and eat.

The hole in the heart is exactly the problem. Even if a man gives me hugs I still crave being touched affectionately, but the problem with men is that physical touch leads to arousal. So I guess that's why I'm stuffing the hole in my heart with food. But it's like a black hole, bottomless. Unfortunately baths, walks, books, music just don't do it for me. They're pleasant enough but the activities are all solo and nothing compares even vaguely to physical touch. I specifically want to feel connected and close to another human being. For the past year I've done creative movement which involved being very intimate with other bodies and that was incredible. The amount of kindness & nurturing I felt turned it into a spiritual experience for me.

When women feel 'connected', their feel-good serotonin-producing factory clicks into high gear and life feels good. However, what qualifies as a sense of connectivity can keep you searching endlessly. Everything in our culture would have us believe it is essential to have a romantic relationship, when often other forms of connection can be just as valuable. You needn't downgrade them purely because they aren't of the romantic kind. The problem is, if you become fixated on having a particular type of relationship, everything else pales in comparison so you wander around, forever feeling unfulfilled and lacking on the inside. This can easily translate into eating to fill from the outside.

What many of us often seek in our relationships is that ecstatic first-time feeling of falling in love or lust. Problem is, ecstasy happens briefly, but just like the drug with the same name, you land up craving that feeling permanently. Happiness and contentment, in comparison with ecstasy, appear dull and insufficient to being 'over the moon'. The problem isn't insufficient ecstasy. It's confusing ecstasy with happiness, and believing that's the permanent feeling you need to have. Aim for a life that comes with big chunks of contentment and serenity, substantial blocks of happiness, and spikes of delicious ecstasy. Self-love is recognising that what you are most seeking is the sense of connection with your Essential Self and the feeling of being energetically connected to others.

Hope

> Now you'd think that Hope is a positive thing to have – but in my case it's what constantly sabotages me. Every time a new diet hits the shelves, I'm first to buy it. I swear I've tried every diet ever created. Finally, though, I've started to see this pattern for what it is – one that can never work. Feeling hopeful about yet another diet, or another handful of pills, is like believing a spider's web won't break if I walk through it.

Hope is an ingredient that Diet City gurus are most invested in keeping alive because that's what keeps Dietonians hooked. But when we learn to rely on our own internal resources, we don't need to be told by external advisors how to run our bodies.

There comes a time in your life when you finally 'get it', when in the midst of the insanity and the obsessive attempts to change your body, your inner voice cries out 'Enough! Stop!' It usually happens when you've fought and struggled so much you realize there *has* to be a better way, another set of choices. This is when you finally see through the hope promised by bottles, vials or prescriptive eating; you 'get' that being thin is not what living is all about. When it happens it's as if a profound sense of serenity wraps around us. The need to become self-loving overtakes the need to please others. That's when true hope finally catches up with you.

Make a list of all the things you hope for that aren't related in any way to your appearance. What do you hope for emotionally and spiritually? Remember words have power – just writing your hopes creates changes in your body chemistry and makes what you wish for more concrete.

Imperfection

I grew up believing I had to hate myself if I wasn't perfect. It's almost as if, in being harsh and critical of myself, I was showing the world that I was aware I had a problem. And by not doing things, like wearing a swimsuit on the beach or dancing at a disco, I was acknowledging that there was something wrong with me. So at least I wasn't committing the double crime of being fat but also not doing anything about it.

I admit to having been an aspirant perfectionist. I say 'aspirant' because no amount of striving to be perfect ever took me to that place of peacefulness I assumed accompanied being perfect. In fact the harder I tried, the more frantic I became because inner peace and perfectionism aren't comfortable bed partners. When I was striving to be perfect, I focused on everything about me that was wrong or substandard. As there was always plenty to focus on, my franticness rose sky-high. Fortunately, I stumbled onto creating what I call my Donald Duck persona. My Donald-Duck-me is the imperfect side of me. She gets cranky, falters and fumbles, doesn't always say or do the 'right' thing, is inconsistent and not always nice. Having a separate, humorous persona has allowed me to stand slightly apart from the imperfections, to accept them as being human and even to laugh about them – something the perfectionist-I was never able to do. I love shrugging my shoulders with an 'Oops! Guess the Donald Duck me just got in the way again. Sorry!' It silences my inner critic and helps me accept some of my less desirable parts. Also, when I treat them lightly, they often go away. I've even grown to like my quirky Donald Duck me! It's been a helpful disguise during my own escape from Diet City.

We are perfect *because* of our imperfections, as the story of the water-bearer illustrates. He carried two pots of water hanging from a stick across his shoulders. The 'perfect' pot arrived full; the other cracked pot was only half-full. The cracked pot, ashamed of its imperfection, apologised to the water-bearer for being flawed. The water-bearer showed the pot a row of cheerful flowers lining the path and pointed out that he'd used the crack to his advantage. He'd planted flower seeds where water from the cracked pot would spill out and water them daily. 'Without you being the way you are, I would not have been able to pick beautiful flowers to decorate my master's table and bring beauty to his house,' he said.

We're all cracked pots – at least in the eyes of a judgemental culture. Once we acknowledge this, our cracks can be used to beautify our lives. Know that in your weaknesses you find other strengths and also some of your beauty. And in the eyes of the Sacred no-one is a cracked pot.

Imperfect parenting

I come from a single-parent home, where my mother broke her back to ensure that we had all we needed, but it comes with a price attached. My mother is a feeder! She feels that the only way to ensure happiness is to make and serve huge portions, this way she 'knows' she is fulfilling her motherly role. Say 'No, thanks' and she takes huge offence, telling everyone she is not worthy of being a mother! So I eat the food, all of it! Now I know why I overeat when I'm feeling guilty or upset. I eat to try and make things better again.

Next time you visit the home you grew up in, look for any clues as to how your attitudes towards food and appearances originated. What Diet City things do your parents say to you and your children about your body, food and eating? Then acknowledge that they often were instilled according to the needs of well-meaning people who only wanted the best for you. They did only what they knew how to in terms of the conventional knowledge of their time. If you find it difficult to forgive your parents for their imperfect parenting, remember that they in turn were shaped by their own imperfect parents, and so on. You can only aspire to learn from their mistakes and hopefully not repeat them yourself.

Intimacy

There was a time when I felt food was the ONLY good thing in my life. It's almost like I had an intimate love affair with it – it was my sensual pleasure, my everything. I didn't know where I ended and where food began. The point now, though, is that I am no longer in a love affair with food. I am just going through the motions. Habit. Food is not the only good thing in my life. And yet, I can't let go.

I so badly wanted a romantic relationship but I was a hopeless failure in this arena. So food became my lover – we were joined at the lips. I could take it to bed with me, it was always delicious, it never spoke back to me, never criticised and it was always there when I wanted it. It was the perfect substitute for what I felt I couldn't have.

Food might masquerade as the perfect substitute for a partner but it isn't. The crumbs it leaves in your bed are not as problematic as the crumbs of guilt it leaves in your mind. Food is a jealous lover. It'll make sure that as it takes over your life, it will *reduce* your chances of finding the mate you truly desire. Not so much because you're gaining weight, but because you're more likely to feel unattractive and repulsive to yourself. You will then act accordingly and push people away.

Think long term and ask yourself, is spending more time with food really helping me have the kind of relationships that fill and nourish me? Or is it pushing other potential lovers away? Care for yourself enough to make self-loving choices.

Jealousy

My husband was gorgeous and bubbly. Me? I was plain and bulgy. Just the thought that he might find someone else made me eat. The bigger my body became, the more paranoid I became that he would leave me – even though it was me, and never him, that complained about my body. Therapy helped me to see that it was my behaviour (and not my body) that would land up causing the very thing I feared the most – driving him away. I had double standards: I was spending so much of my mental time having an affair with Jealousy and that was robbing my husband and me of having a healthy relationship.

The majority of people love you because of your personality and actions, not because of your appearance. Take a quick look around your friends – why do you like them? Because they're extremely beautiful or because it makes *you* look better having someone nice-looking around? I doubt it! If someone is only with you because of the way you look, you'll be forever insecure, worrying about whether they find someone else with fewer wrinkles, perkier breasts, a firmer tummy or thighs – or just someone prettier than you.

Write down all the friends you have that you would never consider giving up just because they have fat thighs, or a wobbly stomach, or butt that looks like two ferrets fighting in a sack. Write down next to each name what it is you value about them.

Kleptomania

If I was feeling edgy, the dread would start because I knew I'd find myself sussing out which shop I was going to shoplift from. The urge to get rid of that wound-up feeling was so overwhelming. I'd do my stealing and that temporary feeling of omnipotence erased those jittery feelings. Later the remorse came and then I'd eat into oblivion.

Your Essential Self is a beautiful, wonderful person. But there is a little cavity just before you get to the centre of your Essential Self that collects bad thoughts, keeping them separate so they don't taint the honourable parts of you. It's also in this tiny chamber where you live in a jittery state of hope – that someone will help you remember your Sacredness. It's in this tiny room where you know that retail therapy of the unpaid kind and other less honourable deeds aren't really a part of you – and that the person you're robbing is yourself. The centre of your Essential Self feels less safe when your actions are being promoted by that little room. Very often, this little cavity is one of our most secretive places – we keep it hidden in the dark thinking that it would be best if no-one else knew about it. But shining light into dark cavities can often be what highlights the way out. Allowing others to know those secrets is often to discover that you can still be accepted and loved. That's what is healing.

Inadequacy

What has really been an eye-opener for me has been to do thin-fantasies. When I am honest with myself, I see that even in the thin-fantasy, I STILL feel inadequate! It's obviously the inadequacy I have to work on – not the striving for perfection!

It's easier to concentrate on growing self-love than trying to shrink inadequacy. You can feel the difference in power between focusing on: 'What would be a more self-loving action?' versus 'What would be a less inadequate action?' You're immediately drawn towards doing something positive when you think about becoming 'more than' the 'less than' person you were. So, I've gone on a lot about making internal changes. What about exterior ones – can those not be self-loving? Of course they can give you a lift, and also provide you with the impetus to get started on making internal changes that will help you escape Diet City permanently. But shifting your focus towards building your self-esteem and confidence from the inside out, rather than from the exterior, is ultimately what will bring about the most sustainable changes.

Advertisements make claims, either explicitly or by implication, that if we use their product/s, we'll become transformed and look like their models (who in real life seldom use the products they advertise). The basic message is, using their products will change our lives – give us confidence, increase our sense of self-worth, magically dissolve all our self-doubt and inadequacies. However advertisers *need* us to be insecure for us to want their products. It's their job to persuade us there is something inherently flawed in our natural, non-touched-up selves. Okay, so wearing a new brand of lipstick may temporarily make you feel better about yourself. But think about it, it's not the product itself but the effect it has on you internally in changing your own perception of your image. If you can do it with a swish of colour on your lips, you could do it *without* the lipstick too, because it's what you *believe* the lipstick has done to change you that makes the difference. Not the lipstick itself.

Change the focus of how you imagine you'd like to be. Instead of imagining yourself as being skinny, imagine yourself being as confident as you desire, even with the body you have right now. Ask yourself what you'd do differently if you were filled with confidence, then practise living as if that were true.

Insecurity

My family was one filled with high achievers, and I never seemed to reach quite the same level as my siblings. I always felt insecure and hungry for the praise and validation I thought my brothers and sisters always received. Even though my husband gave me lots of praise, no matter how much I got, it never seemed enough. My bingeing was one way of filling myself with 'more than enough'. I've read so many books and been to workshops that have all helped me change those old childhood thoughts of: 'I'm not enough and I can't get enough' to 'I'm enough, I do enough and I have enough.' Now, whenever old feelings intrude I go to my 'treasure box' of cards and letters from people that remind me of my worth, and after spending a few minutes with these gems, the urge to eat seems to dissipate on it's own.

A lack of self-esteem stems from having limiting beliefs about you and it's the biggest hurdle most people face today in their quest for a happy existence. We started as amazing babies full of promise, potential and possibility. Now we're adults with body fears and food hang-ups. What happened? We aren't born with the fear of being inadequate – it happens when our confidence is chipped away.

When I escaped from Diet City, I found it easier to figure out what would bring me a sense of *serenity* rather than a sense of *adequacy*. You see serenity can appear in an instant – if you pause long enough to take in a few deep breaths, you immediately feel more serene – whereas a sense of security takes a lot longer to arrive. If each time you face a choice, and you choose what will bring you serenity, a sense of security will eventually grow out of that.

Collect up valued documents like cards, letters and photos to create your own treasure chest you can dig into. You don't have any? No problem, ask all your friends and family to write you a short note about what it is they most appreciate or like about you. Then when you feel insecure, instead of turning to food, turn your feet firmly in the direction of your treasure chest.

Instant gratification

My husband's late stepmother was an anorexic and a bulimic – even at 69! She looked like an Auschwitz survivor. Her methods of weight control were extreme, the vomit/laxative/diuretic route – she was taking no chances! She had numerous collapses and finally ended up in ICU. She never put an end to her deadly habits, but they put an end to her. As desperate as I am to lose these dratted pounds I watched my stepmother-in-law's progress with increasing revulsion over the years and if ever there was a warning not to try pills that was it.

I went through a period of my life when I swallowed a daily cocktail of appetite suppressants, laxatives and sometimes diuretics as well. It's a sad indictment of a health system that sold those kinds of products to a young girl barely out of her teens! I was hooked – not only on the products but what I thought they could do for me: help me lose weight effortlessly, turbo-fast.

Today's technology allows e-mails and SMS's to fly across cyberspace in milliseconds. We live in a faster, bigger, better, wanting-more-NOW society which has made us increasingly impatient. We can't be content with a slower Internet connection when there's an even faster one just comes on the market. Ironically, the places on our planet where the pace of life has sped up the most through modern technology also have the fattest people. We seldom walk anywhere; there are even have moving sidewalks at airports to speed us up. For many families, meals prepared from raw ingredients have been shelved in favour of more convenient pre-packaged meals or drive-thrus or take-outs. Sitting down to savor a single meal in a day is a challenge. We eat on the run, we don't get enough rest; life is like being on a giant whirling Ferris wheel.

In terms of dieting, if the quick-weight loss pills don't do the trick, there is the more instant plastic surgery method. Escaping Diet City means giving up on these supposed instant gratification methods. Weight that comes off too quickly rebounds twice as fast. It is much healthier to lose the weight more slowly and over a longer period of time, not only so your body can make adjustments but so that your mind can too.

Each day, take time out to do something beautiful slowly. Sit in your garden doing nothing except feeling the sun on your face or listening to the sounds around you. Take time out to examine the beauty of a dandelion, leaf or an intricate flower. Leave enough time for you to enjoy an extended bath or to drive to your destination at a leisurely pace and revel in how good it feels to let your body rhythms slow down.

Loneliness

When we got divorced after 25 years of marriage, food became my time-filler. Then I started going to a weekly support group for divorcees. On those evenings I came back feeling uplifted and motivated. On those nights it never occurred to me to eat. I realized how quickly an evening could pass when I was excited about something. I started doing some baby-sitting and somehow being in someone else's home didn't leave me feeling empty and alone. When I saw this, I also knew it was time to sell up the home that had always been 'ours' and buy a smaller place that I could make 'mine.' When the last packed box left our shared home, I felt like I'd taken a big step towards reclaiming my life.

Learn to keep good company with yourself. Make sure your own company is of a high quality – if you turn to food when you're lonely, it's only a misguided way of not being alone. But the company you're usually left with is Discomfort and Guilt. Take yourself out on a date or to a movie (we don't have to wait for people to come to us), or invite others in. Just because you are alone, doesn't mean you have to be lonely. We are fabulous even by ourselves.

Living large

I'm extremely afraid of alienating people. I think it's because as a kid I was told that being myself was what pushed people away from me. I was always told to tone it down. I learned to hate the child I was - I've learned to shun her as a total social freak with no grace and no humility: a spaz. I use food to suppress my potential, continuously eating too much. It's almost like I'm terrified to fit into my personality because it seems much bigger than my physical body. If we go to a party, I want to be there in the thick of things shaking my body – but I'm much too fearful of getting out there, letting myself go and making an ass of myself because I've danced myself into my personality. My greatest challenge is acknowledging that it's okay to live a life the size I deserve.

What is the life that suits you? Is living larger than life the real you or is it a mask for feeling insufficient? When it's the latter, you feel empty because the life you're living is a backstage one – the one people don't see. And when you really do have a large personality but you downplay your wonderful, enthusiastic self so that people only see a suppressed version, you thirst for an authentic life.

When you live a life that doesn't fit you, you're so busy being on- or off-stage that you often don't see that in the larger scheme of things, you are richer than you could ever dream. How much would you give for your sight? Your hearing? Your friends? And even daily hassles, like hating those thighs? Remember only those who are dead and buried don't have issues.

Make an inventory of all your assets – and don't downplay them with 'if only' or 'buts'.

When you turn up the volume on life – living whatever personality really suits you – life feels sweeter. For the life you're living to fit your personality, what parts of yourself do you need to expand or shrink? Of a flamboyant or a quiet personality, none is better than the other. They are simply different, and the world needs both. I once read something by Neil Donald Walsh (author of *Conversations with God*) where he admitted that many of the personal characteristics he'd been criticised for were actually wonderful characteristics, just with the volume turned up too high. His outspokenness reflected a willingness to speak his mind – but a little too forcefully. Therefore, what he needed to do was not get rid of those character traits, but learn to use only as much of the trait as was required for each situation. When you feel that the personality the world sees is the authentic you, you've taken a major step away from life in Diet City.

Make a list of the personal character traits that trouble you or that you have been criticised for. On which would you like to turn the volume up or down?

Loss of identity

I was made redundant two weeks ago. Whoa! In flooded fear, upset, panic, etc. I no longer have a job became 'but I do still have food, and for as long as I have it let me eat it because if I don't get another job I might not have food either.' This made me realize how unbalanced my life was: all about my job and food and nothing else.

When you live an unbalanced life and something happens to tilt your world so that the way you mainly define yourself falls away, it's the Universe giving you a nudge. It's forcing you to re-evaluate and make important changes.

The moment life becomes difficult and you aren't getting what you think you want or need, it's tempting to wonder what you've done to deserve this or why your Creator did this to you. It's not that you're being punished, it is simply life unfurling. On the surface life might appear to be unfair; bad things happen to good people and sometimes individuals who commit heinous deeds seem to get off scot-free.

You will never know the full story. When you're in the midst of difficulties, it's helpful to remind yourself that, even though it may not feel like it, life is unfolding exactly as it should in order to present each of you with precisely the opportunities you need to grow.

Getting thin may feel really fabulous, but it may also be what brings on problems of infertility or osteoporosis later on in life. Not being able to lose the pounds you've regained could be just what you need to develop those parts of your personality that might otherwise have stayed dormant and undiscovered. You may consider the job you lost a tragedy when in fact it ends up opening new and exciting doors for you. Think about this scenario: you land up missing your aeroplane for a vitally important business trip, which means you're likely to get fired. Very unlucky. But what if the plane crashed? What at first seemed terribly unlucky becomes *very* lucky.

Difficulties may tempt you into becoming engulfed in negativism. But if you choose to acknowledge and celebrate the fact that one door *never* closes without another opening, you clear the way for the Universe to present you with all sorts of unexpected surprises. If you obscure that doorway with panic and fear, you blind yourself to the opportunities sitting right under your nose. One of the amazing things about being in Nature's Valley is being able to see that what at first appears to be a disaster is actually an opportunity hiding out in the rough. It's not just about taking lemons and turning them into lemonade. It's realizing that your life has the potential to *improve* because of the lemons themselves.

Lying

Lying has kept me out of trouble but it has got to a point where not even my closest friends trust me anymore. I'm so caught up in lies that I have to tell new lies to hide the previous lies. The other day, my school counsellor pulled me aside. Instead of shouting at me for lying about food I'd taken from the staffroom, she hugged me with real compassion and asked if I'd ever considered that all I was doing by lying was trying to hide parts of myself I

We weren't born liars. It was only as we grew up, we discovered that telling the whole truth got us into trouble and that embroidering the truth resulted in positive strokes. It can be difficult to stop lying when telling the truth while you were growing up had harsh consequences. Lying is an indication that you don't feel safe enough or confident enough in the reactions of others or you don't have enough confidence in yourself. Taking the more challenging option will stand you in good stead because intentions – good or bad – are energy. Your thoughts are energy; for this reason, both parties are affected by a lie, even when only one of you knows about it.

Much of living in Diet City is one big lie. Advertisers lie; gorgeous models are photo-enhanced lies and scales lie about your self-worth. You lie to yourself when you decide you can only be happy once your body looks a certain way. Start shedding those lies and, buried underneath, you'll find the truth. You will be happy not once your body changes but when you believe you *deserve* to be happy. You're already fabulous exactly as you are.

When you're tempted to lie, ask yourself what you're trying to avoid or get more of? What is it about the particular situation or person you're tempted to lie to that's tripping you up? Resolve to become spiritually honest. In being spiritually honest you're being truthful and in harmony with the Universe.

Motherhood

Eating was the one way I could have 'my' share, put myself first. It was the one way I felt I could 'mother' myself. Ironically motherhood provided the trigger for my overeating, and I became a really bad role model. But in the end it also helped me to stop it. When my son came home from school one day with a note to say that he was obese, I realized how desperately I didn't want him to be fat or teased. My motivation to prevent this was so strong that eating healthier and exercising for his sake became quite easy.

The physical pain of labour pales into insignificance by comparison to the pain mothers experience when their child is being teased or hurt. Being a mother forever changes your vulnerabilities and your priorities, finely honing your protective instincts. When you're a mother, escaping Diet City takes on a new urgency. As a mother, in becoming motivated to help your child, you can accomplish what you would otherwise find difficult to do for yourself simply to help your child escape pain and suffering.

Neglect

I grew up in a children's home where love and food were in short supply. I grew up thinking that when food was available you ate as much as possible because you never knew when it would be available again. Even though I married into 'the jet set' and had money to buy good nutritious food, I didn't. In many ways I neglected myself as much as the nuns did in my childhood. Two years ago, at a friend's birthday, she had a chef come to her house. Her party was one big cooking extravaganza. I loved the care that went into the way he prepared his food and signed up for cooking lessons with him. Now I place more emphasis on the quality than the quantity of food I'm eating. The care that goes into my healthy food preparation is a tangible way of caring for me.

If we could objectively view our lives, we'd see that part of being trapped in Diet City is being trapped in the Valley of negative Echoes. When you look in the mirror and your internal critic shouts, 'I hate you!', that self-hatred boomerangs back to you. If you shout out, 'I love you!' self-love will bounce back at you. If you want to have more love, gentleness and respect, then *radiate* out more those qualities, not just to others but to yourself as well. That is what life will deliver back to your doorstep. Life is a mirror of what you put out there – you create and manifest your own reality with your thoughts, actions and intentions.

To change the negatives that life is echoing back to you, stop hating your body unless you want body hatred to grow. Leaving Diet City is leaving the Valley of negative Echoes. When you reach Nature's Valley life will give back to you something completely different. As Gandhi said, 'Be the change you want to see in the world.' When you change yourself – your thoughts and actions – your reality will change too.

Want to leave the Valley of negative Echoes? Remember that your brain can't tell the difference between what is real and what isn't.

Choose positive affirmations and even if you don't initially believe in them, say them over and over. You can make up your own affirmations. Start them with 'I' and make sure they affirm what you wish for – but as if you already have it. The more you repeat your affirmations, the more you're building that neural pathway. Use the following affirmations (or adapt them): I live in harmony with my body; I am at peace with my being; I live a healthy, happy, wholesome life.

Passion-less

My 'change your body, change your life' programming began at a very early age and has been almost impossible to get rid of. My life's energy hasn't gone towards anything worthwhile. Instead, I've hated my body and tried to change it through either over-exercising or under-eating and, of course, comparing myself to 20-year-old models when I'm a 35-year-old mother of four. If I died right now, all I'd have to show for it is self-loathing. Is that the kind of legacy I want to leave my children?

When I ask Mind over Fatter pilgrims to plot their weight line, their weight-worry line and their passion-for-life line on a graph, I see an interesting pattern. When passion goes up, weight and weight-worry diminish. This is exactly why living a life of passion and purpose is a powerful light illuminating the path to Nature's Valley.

When you focus your life's energy on trivialities, you've forgotten that your life is an expression of Divine purpose and energy. Feeling wonder-filled about life is what you get when you live fully. Living a less than passionate life is a cop-out because you've been gifted with talents and abilities – special qualities only you can use in the way you do. Depending on you, these gifts are enhanced or lessened. If you choose to live a life with passion – even without any pay – the rewards of feeling alive, valued and filled with worth are remuneration enough. (This doesn't mean you can't get paid for your passions – if you can find a way to make them income-producing, drum rolls and applause for you!)

Many of us are searching for our 'purpose in life' as though it's a single, clear-cut thing – but we're searching 'out there' instead of 'in here'. Some of us go wandering off to foreign lands thinking we'll discover our passion there, when the only journey we need to make is one back to that Essential Self. Some people find their passions evolve from the ashes of hardship. They're driven to prevent others from experiencing what they did. Others are driven by positive experiences because they want others to share what they've been through.

So you think you don't know what you're passionate about? Sift through past hopes and dreams, the systems you believe in and value, the loyalties and affections you've gained from people you love (and those who love you) to find the values you hold dear. When you use them as the central focus to guide you into action, you'll soon remember what you're passionate about.

Make a graph of your weight line, your weight-worry line and your passion-for-life line. What about your weight stands out for you when you compare the times you've been excited about life with the times you haven't?

Perfectionism

The more I strove for perfection, the less in control I felt and the more out of control my eating became. I may have been fooling others, but I could no longer fool myself. My perfectionist standards were exhausting and the goal posts kept moving. Dropping ridiculous standards was what was needed, not trying ever harder to become more perfect.

One of the things I felt my weight was saying was that it was protecting me from self-hatred. So I started a journal. And what came out was that, as long as I'm overweight, I've got something to blame for not being perfect. If I were thin and still not perfect, then that would mean there was an intrinsic fault in me. That completely floored me!

If you're out of balance somewhere else in your life and it's showing up in your eating, correct the imbalance – and the eating will usually correct itself. Out-of-whack eating is often your body's way of fighting to maintain balance in a world that seems overly ordered and sterile. Striving for perfection is so limiting. It is limiting of joy, of creativity and of having a fun-filled life. When perfectionism is in the driving seat and you're busy trying to be perfect, everyone else is busy living life, laughing and having fun. So strive away if you have to but just think: wouldn't it be much more fun and wouldn't you feel vastly more alive if you painted, planted or played? Don't waste time while there are rainbows to chase, rivers to swim, ideas to fly with, and a full and varied life to lead. It's hard to be young at heart (which is where it counts) and impossibly perfect all at once.

Ironically, the less attached you are to things being perfect, the more chance you have of feeling like a winner. Are you a winner because your house is dust-free or because you're living a full life, albeit with the odd cobweb in your home? There's really no need to strive incessantly to get rid of the imperfections. Defending picky, perfectionist ways only proves that you are perfectly imperfect – because you're allowing perfectionism to control you. Relax, and strive instead to become more comfortable with imperfection. That's a first step out of Diet City.

How would your life change if you were no longer driven to achieve particular body size or eating standards? Pretend that you've been spirited away by forces to a land where expectations of achieving any particular standards are totally gone. Are there cells in your body that would sigh a happy release from the fear and panic-related neuropeptides that have been overloading your system?

Protection

> *My fat is my protection, it makes people feel safe. I love that my friends will leave me alone with their husbands, knowing they are perfectly safe. I don't want to lose the fat because I'm scared of who I'd become if I lost this part of me. It's like, better the fat-devil I know than the thin one I'm too scared to uncover.*

Insulating yourself from life with additional layers is like keeping a wild bird in a cage. The cage may well keep predators at bay – but at what cost? And is this a cost you're willing to pay? You may feel it protects you from yourself and others, but how about the ways it keeps you from spreading your wings? And if you never get a chance to spread those wings, you'll also never get a chance to strengthen them and soar to great heights. Much better protection would be to strengthen trust that you have the ability to deal with whatever life puts in your path. Trust that you can emerge from your shell, escape that body cage, and live more lightly.

If you were to let yourself believe that the world was a safe place for just 30 seconds, what might present itself to you that you're not seeing while hiding behind those extra layers? Is it possible that you might find a new vision of yourself and the world?

Rebellion

> *At Sunday lunches, we always had yummy roast potatoes. One Sunday, I decided to have a second helping. I'd only intended taking one when my aunt leaned across, put her fork on my outstretched hand and said: 'Darling, you don't really need that second helping, do you?' Inside my head I could clearly hear myself going, one potato, two potatoes, three potatoes ... four! and then taking three more than I'd planned to. It may sound dumb – after all whom was I hurting, for heaven's sake? But it was my way of rebelling against being controlled. Ironically, by choosing a response that ultimately hurt me, I was allowing my aunt to control my eating ... in a different way. Once I had that figured, I started a new kind of rebellion by insisting on doing only what I really wanted – like eating only one – instead of reacting to oppose others.*

> *My husband nags me about my weight (he says he doesn't). Don't get me wrong, he's not a bad guy and he could be thinner himself but he comes from a family where thin is the ultimate. I don't like being told what to do, so my compulsive eating could be a rebellious thing.*

Knowing what you *should* do is one thing but the execution of it is another thing entirely. At some point, though – and this can take a while – you start to feel the internal power of making choices and putting into motion changes in your life. You begin to see the cause and effect of old choices; you 'get it' that new choices bring better results.

In a peculiar kind of way, your large (or small) body can become a monument to you standing up for yourself against the feeling of being controlled. You have the choice to shape your 'monument' in other ways. To really be in control of your eating, you need to decide independently of others what, when and how much you put into your body. If you give away your power to someone who is annoying you, you also prevent yourself from leaving Diet City because you're dancing to their tune instead of your own.

So you don't like being controlled? Good for you! Now stop using this admirable trait in a way that will sabotage you. Instead use your strength to stand up for yourself in a positive way. Ask yourself, how can I rebel in a healthy way? How do I rebel against dieting by refusing to diet? Do I rebel against the belief that implies I'm only lovable and worthwhile dependent on my appearance?

Rejection

> *My husband and I were going through some difficulties. Then one night when I tried to initiate sex, he squirmed away. I felt totally rejected. I got out of bed and wolfed down a whole tub of ice-cream. That he turned me down spoke volumes. I sat there saying hateful things about myself and my body. Eventually I confided in a friend who helped me realize that his turning away might have had nothing to do with me or my body. It might just have been that he didn't feel like sex and felt safe enough with me to 'say' so. Maybe he was having some difficulties of his own at work or maybe it was a symptom for something else he wasn't able to talk about.*

Recently I hiked with a hiking group. My husband was lagging behind and I thought I'd wait for and walk with him, but he kept holding back. I felt upset and hurt that he didn't want to walk with me. But then I watched him more closely and realized he'd slipped into one of those quietly contemplative, meditative spaces. It wasn't that he didn't want my company; he simply wanted to be on his own. It was an important distinction for me to make – that he wasn't rejecting me, rather he was choosing to be present with himself.

So someone suggests a new low-fat product worth trying and we 'hear' them saying we're overweight and need to go on diet. It's not the experience that's the problem, it's the *interpretation* we give the experience. Often we choose the most hurtful motives for people's actions when there are so many other possible explanations. Choosing to interpret a motive as harmful is what causes your anguish and your feelings of being rejected. This gives you one more reason to 'eat it' better. So, try to give others the benefit of the doubt. That way you don't create a reason to turn to comfort eating.

If you're feeling rejected, step back and suspend what you think you 'know' about the situation. Be prepared to accept that someone's motivation may be entirely different to what you have automatically assumed. Take just three minutes to write down as many possible (even if they feel implausible) alternative explanations for their actions. How does it work for you when you choose the explanation on your list that allows you to make a 180-degree change to your feelings? Would it bring you a sense of calm to replace the previous anguish?

Resentment

My own brother conned me out of my inheritance and has walked away scot-free. I'm filled with resentment. Drinking or eating are the only things that seem to keep my resentment down to manageable levels.

I love Neil Donald Walsch's book *The Little Soul and the Sun*. It tells the story of how every soul was created as a perfect light, all part of the greater light. However, in order for a soul to be able to experience its specialness (kind, gentle and forgiving), it needed to be able to experience the dark. For just as warmth cannot be known without cold, light can also not be known without darkness. Since every soul is pure light, in order for darkness to exist another soul has to agree to become something it isn't (the dark). It achieves this by doing something bad not 'to' but 'for' the other soul.

What I love about this perspective is that in reconceptualising bad things being done 'for' us rather than 'against' us, there are no victims or villains - no-one against whom to harbour resentment (a low-energy attractor pattern). It frees us because non forgiveness is a heavy burden. Worst of all, it's like acid that ruins the container holding it; it hurts you at a cellular level. From this perspective, resentment can only exist when the soul on the receiving end of darkness forgets that some soul has merely given up its purity to *benefit* the receiver. When a person appears to have done something bad, it is our duty to continue to be the light as a reminder to the now-dark soul that it, too, was once created in perfect light.

I think of Amy Biehl [30] and how, in the midst of their intense pain and anguish, her parents were able to see that their daughter's murderers had forgotten they once were created as Sacred beings of pure light. Amy's parents were able to direct forgiveness and love (light) to these young men instead of bitterness and resentment (dark). Their pure actions allowed these men to remember their own light. Today, in addition to the light shone by the Biehls, these one-time murderers are projecting their own light. Who knows what powerful impact this is having within their crime-ridden communities?

Do whatever it takes to release yourself from resentment, otherwise it sticks in your throat and will harm you. When you suppress resentment with food, you're not dealing with the real issue and you'll eat your way into permanent residency in Diet City.

Use any bitterness you might feel to drive you into doing something you feel passionate about. Start a web page or an online group for people who have found themselves in a similar situation. Write a book about it for others to learn from. Change your perceptions of the event. How might this help you grow?

Self-doubt

> *I was the youngest and smallest in my class. My parents were forever reminding me that it was okay if I couldn't manage things that other kids could. My mother would do homework for me which I took to mean that I couldn't be trusted to do it well enough myself. My parents were forever rescuing and protecting me, treating me as if I was fragile. I grew up doubting myself; I never developed the trust in my abilities to manage on my own. I couldn't even trust myself around food, because they were forever correcting the times I ate, what I ate and how I ate. When I went to University, I had no-one to regulate my eating and I ballooned. I felt at sea with no parents to guide my every move. I had a really great roommate who refused to 'baby' me. Whenever I said I didn't trust myself to do something, she'd say, 'Nonsense, of course you can!' She was right – I could.*

Whether you think you can or whether you think you can't – either way you are correct, Henry Ford famously once said. That is to say, whatever you personally believe are your abilities, the Universe conspires to get behind you and prove you right. When you first start doing something new, it's natural to have your doubts and feel a bit unsure, but once you push through that self-doubt, you give yourself the opportunity to master things and build your self-belief. This doesn't mean everything will always pan out the way you'd like them to. And when it doesn't, it isn't proof that you can't have a healthy body or you can't live without being dictated to by your scale. No-one gets everything right the first time around. This is especially true of Diet City, where you've tried countless pills, powders, potions and eating plans and had them all fail you. When you're on that path to Nature's Valley, instead of feeling helpless each time you don't get it right; restart the process with the wisdom gleaned from the previous time it occurred. And remember, you are what you believe. If you believe you're out of control around food, you will be. If you believe you cannot trust yourself to make good decisions, then you'll most likely end up making ones that don't seem to work out. You all have the ability to escape Diet City. Even if it sounds like nonsense, keep on saying it until it becomes your truth.

We were all born believing we could achieve anything. It was a truth deep within us. Feelings of doubt come from internalising surface beliefs, then making these lies your truth. Make a list of all the doubts you have about your abilities to leave Diet City and start each of them with the words, 'I believe I can't….' Look at the entire list and note that the only part that's a lie is the 't'. Now go back through the list, crossing the apostrophe and 't' off each sentence. Read them first thing in the morning and last thing at night.

Selfishness

> *My recently widowed mother has moved in with us. It sounds so selfish to say this, but I'm tired of mothering her. I feel so weary and emptied out by mothering both her and my two small children – the only way I feel I can get any sustenance to 'mother' is through eating.*
>
> *I have trouble discerning the difference between selfish and self-nurturing. We've grown up in a society that idolises the woman who is always giving to others without any thought of herself – and demonises the woman trying to meet her own needs (even when she is meeting the needs of everyone else around her!). How warped is that? So, a lot of what I'm going through is fighting these old, ingrained, disordered beliefs and forging my own new path in life.*

Imagine how ridiculous it would be if you always insisted on putting another's needs ahead of your own? 'No, we must eat your diet food, that's what you want.' 'No, but I insist, you want a banquet, that's what we will have.' You'd forever be going around in circles with a lot of individuals not having their needs met. Women have a much harder time putting their own needs first because of our still-prevalent conditioning to be nurturers and caretakers who are always there for others. We've followed our mother role-models, who learnt from their mother role-models. And of course we've watched our father role-models (who in turn learned from their fathers) expecting to have their needs met. It doesn't come naturally to put our needs first so we've become used to putting feelings of entitlement aside, and we constantly forfeit our own needs.

Women yearn to lighten the load imposed by societal expectations (surface truths). You have as much right as men do to want things for yourself – that's not selfishness. To accomplish this, you need to move away from fear-based submission towards a self-respecting assertion. This is possible when you believe you deserve to be treated with kindness, honour and respect. It's the truth from deep within. Also, if you only put the needs of others ahead of yours all the time, you run the risk of burn-out. Your spirit will be diminished until your life is governed, not by the person you truly are but by a person driven by resentment and anger. Leaving Diet City entails growing in such a way that you are no longer prepared to settle for less than what you're entitled to.

Make preserving the person you'd like to be a higher priority than doing everything for others. Remind yourself that it is not selfish to learn to say a self-respecting 'No'. If not, you may well struggle to say 'No' to food as well, for it will simply mirror back to you what's going on elsewhere in your life.

Self-hatred

My large body was the blanket I wrapped around my self hatred. My 'blanket' needed to be so large because there was so much self-hatred needing to be wrapped.

Let's cradle and rock those parts of ourselves that we're convinced are so unlovable, and watch how doing this can help them soften and transform. Remember that mind makes matter – so it really is Mind over Fatter. Self-love can literally melt away the fat mentality that keeps us in Diet City.
Read and reread the chapter on self-love (Chapter Five).

Secrets

> *As long as I could keep my body's imperfections clearly in focus, or concentrate on what exercise routine was best and how well I was doing it, or I had a diet to follow and could focus on how well I was following it, I didn't have to deal with other more painful issues. Keeping my mouth full kept me from talking about the incest I carried such deep shame about. I joined a wonderful group of other incest survivors where I realized that my father didn't abuse me because of some lack within me, but because of a sense of power within himself that he was missing. I was a courageous survivor and not a helpless victim. The night I told my story, I left that meeting room feeling like I'd shed some sort of an unclean skin and with that some old eating habits went as well.*
>
> *My secret eating was masking the other secret I was hiding: that I'm gay. How could I tell my husband, children and my parents? They would be shocked and it would hurt so many people. Through online conversations with other married gay women, I realized I wasn't alone. When my twins finished school, I told my children who didn't seem as devastated as I thought they would be so long as I wasn't going to embarrass them. My husband and parents were devastated, but after being honest I felt like I'd shed pounds.*

Keeping a secret gives it the power to grow into a monster. Because you only have yourself to bounce ideas on, what really happens is a repetitive going around and around of the same confusing issues. This only leads to growing isolation and self-doubt. By never sharing your secret, you don't allow in alternative information that could shine light into the darkness. Using food, talk of diets or your own performance to distract yourself from a painful secret can work for a short, temporary while but such dark secrets can also stop you from living a light and bright life.

Do you feel safer walking in the sunshine or walking after dark? Isn't it true that when the light is shining, things often seem less ominous? Think about it this way: you're unlikely to be the only person who has experienced whatever it is you're feeling shameful about. When you link up with others who share parts of your story, what you're hiding seems less shameful and you can feel supported and cared for in ways you might never have expected.

Ask yourself this: What parts of me am I finding unacceptable? What parts of me am I so ashamed of that I feel I have to hide? When you find out what they are, work on them rather than on the eating itself.

84

Sexual attention

I remember the day I started eating – I was eight. It was the day my sixteen-year-old brother walked into my room, pulled my panties off and put his fingers inside of me. These times confused me. I loved that he wanted to show me how much he loved me, but it terrified me. My large body became my armor; it made me feel less exposed. Even after my brother stopped, I kept eating. As long as I had my large body, I didn't have to risk opening myself up to a relationship. I thought I wanted to lose weight so I went on every diet imaginable. But every time I started attracting sexual attention, I'd sabotage myself.

Trauma of this nature becomes encoded in your cellular memory. There are many therapies that could work for you to help you physically release those traumatic memories at a cellular level; look for one that resonates with you.

Do you like to talk? Then try a psychologist. Do you love to dance? Join up for dance or movement therapy. Do you like to draw? Art might be your therapy. Do you find writing therapeutic? Write your own story looking for strengths in your personality that might have developed from the trauma. Do your dreams remind you of the trauma? Working with the symbols from your dreams may help. Or there's massage, reiki, crystal healing or a multiplicity of other complementary health modalities.

Stepping into yourself

I was going for a job at an advertising agency –I knew I'd be by far the largest person there, and not just by a little bit either. But I also had great skills. I figured I wasn't going to get the job because of my looks. I bought a new outfit that I felt good in, I walked taller, I put a smile into my voice and on my face and thought, What the heck, I might as well enjoy myself, I'm just going to have fun. I let my funny side loose, I was sassy and I teased my interviewees outrageously. It was like I really stepped into myself and allowed myself to be all aspects of my personality. I'd just made a mental note to fake it but after a while I wasn't faking it. My body language said: Love me or leave me. They loved me. They hired me.

I remember when I finally came out of my phase of hating myself and said to my husband, 'You hated me when I was fat.' He replied, 'It never made any difference to me whether you were fat or thin. What did make a difference was how you changed when you thought you were fat. You wouldn't change or get undressed in front of me and you pushed me away every time I wanted to touch you.' How you feel about yourself has less to do with your body than it has to do with what is going on in your *mind*. When you become comfortable with you, regardless of whether your body has changed or not, you also change how you act and react.

'People are like stained-glass windows – they sparkle and shine when the sun is out, but when the darkness sets in, their true beauty is revealed only if there is a light within.' (Elizabeth Kubler-Ross) That light lurking within is the sense of joy we once were so in touch with as children. Joy and lightness are wonderful potions to pack in your lunchbox when leaving Diet City, for they can be your guiding stars whenever you feel like you may have lost the path. When you let your personality out of its hiding place, it changes what people see about you. They no longer 'see' your bulges; what draws them to you is your spunky spirit, your great sense of humour and sense of fun. They see someone who can enrich their lives, someone who they'd like to have around. It's not your body that's ever really the problem; it's your relationship with it. Sometimes you have to find ways to sidestep yourself, to get out of your own way.

Ask yourself: What do I need to do right now, this minute, to be more joyful and light, to let more of my personality shine through? Then follow what it is, so that it can light your way.

Uniqueness

Being able to read other people's online posts was so calming for me – it's unbelievable how all of us had such very similar struggles. But it also had an unexpected aspect to it. The more I read everyone's entries, the more I realized that my struggles weren't that unique or anything special. The fact that this made me feel sad instead of glad told me that there was something about my food and body oddities that gave me a sense of being unique and different. It was these issues that were adding value to my life!

The great thing about realizing how important a sense of uniqueness is to you is that it opens up other possibilities for you to explore in terms of other sides to your uniqueness – aspects that you value and want to honour. It allows you to think of ways you might like to express yourself other than eating.

You wouldn't want people to remember you for the uniqueness of your food and body oddities, so find ways to expand your fabulous uniqueness such that they release you from Diet City rather than keeping you from leaving it.

Fast forward your life to a 'remembering ceremony' that might be held on your deathbed by people who know and love you. If they were commenting on all the unique, special and different qualities they'd noticed about you, what would you like them to be commenting on?

Victimhood

I had an awful childhood in which 'poor me' became a part of my identity. I could always find someone to blame for everything that went wrong in my life. I was the victim. 'Poor me' feelings were followed by 'feed me', which inevitably led to 'fat me' and became 'unhappy me'. The unhappier I became, the more I blamed my circumstances and the people in my life. It became a vicious cycle that only started improving when I reminded myself that as an adult, I could either be a part of the problem or a part of the solution.

It may seem as if others are the problem. If only *they* would change, you wouldn't get so angry. But the only way to change others is to change yourself, your actions and reactions. No-one else can force you to be angry and no-one else can take your feelings away – those are choices *you* make.

When you hold onto victimhood, you trap emotional energy that could be used far more positively. Rather use your energy to affirm and love life. It's a lack of forgiveness that keeps you stuck with a victim-identity. Instead, try claiming the identity of someone who forgives. Even if that person doesn't appear to deserve forgiveness, forgiving affirms the goodness that is inherently a part of you. Forgiveness is like sterilising a wound, which allows healing and releases energy for growth. Don't hold back on being forgiving 'until the other person apologises' or 'justice has been served.' That's holding onto a life filled with mental prison bars of bitterness. Remember, you're the one being sentenced, not the other person (who may not even be aware they have hurt you). I love American psychologist and talk show host Phil McGraw's idea of forgiveness, where he says it's about releasing yourself from giving someone else the ability to make your heart turn cold and to be less of the person you'd like to be.

Take a tip from the legend of an Indian chief, whose village had just been attacked, leaving a trail of devastation. He said to his grandson, 'Right now I have two wolves fighting in my heart. One wolf wants vengeance and is urging me to retaliate and kill. The other wolf wants peace and is urging me to forgive.' 'Which of the two wolves will win, Grandfather?' asked the boy curiously. 'The wolf that I feed, said the wise old man.

Whenever you find yourself thinking, *you* made me feel....' change it to, 'I choose to feel....' In this way you will acknowledge your power and take responsibility for your feelings. This way you choose growing better over growing bitter.

Worthlessness

It was time to step out: break my celibacy, make more of an effort with my appearance and generally enjoy who I am. When I met someone I thought I'm making progress. The man told me I'm 'not his physical ideal' which I have used as an excuse to punish myself for being FAT, a monster, a failure, and so on, and of course also a wonderful excuse to eat. The question is: why do I attempt to get involved with someone who so clearly doesn't appreciate me? I fear the answer is that I still, despite a six-year abstinence and lots of work on myself, choose men who confirm to me that I'm not worthy – firstly by getting involved with Mr Wrong (again!), secondly by giving his words such power, and thirdly by sticking to old, useless behaviour – eating. Comfort eating will not solve my problems; it's part of my outdated behaviour that no longer serves me.

If you keep repeating unhelpful behaviour such as eating badly, not doing things you really like, not believing you deserve better, not leaving situations in which you feel dishonoured, not trusting your inner wisdom, or not having relationships you would find fulfilling, then maybe you don't believe that you deserve the best self-care possible. Start building a new sense of self-worth. Remember that you reflect your feelings of inadequacy back at yourself. Feelings of unworthiness manifest as behaviours that only *confirm* your lack of worthiness.

Do just one thing each day this week to help you appreciate the worthiness of *you*!

As these morsels illustrate, dieting doesn't get to the heart of the matter, to the 'why' of eating. We often feel simultaneously starving and stuffed – full yet still empty. We subject ourselves to ongoing attempts to change ourselves into something the media and models (so thin you can fax them) espouse as *the* way to attain happiness, only to find that yo-yo dieting leaves us even hungrier on the inside. The reason for this? What is needed is *mind* rather than body remodelling – and this takes time, patience and persistence because the mind works in convoluted ways. It's not the changes to our bodies that make us great. It's the changes we make to our minds.

Chapter 4:

♥

Thinland –is it a Happy Place?

We pursue the illusion that happiness and fulfilment arrive on the doorstep just as soon as a specific number on the scale does too. Unless you have changed your internal view of yourself, this won't happen in any long term way. This is why The Joy-Filled Body is a journey to the mentally, spiritually and physically rich place called Nature's Valley, not another march to Thinland. Thinland is the Land of Oz, a mythical place of smoke and mirrors where Dietonians imagine everything is perfect so long as their weight is. Of course, no-one ever really gets there because, well, frankly merely changing your body doesn't impact on your Essential Self. Instead, your fruitless striving only gets you stuck deeper in Diet City. It may surprise you to know that 'thin and happy' don't necessarily belong in the same sentence. *My mental images did not alter with the weight loss, and I found it extremely difficult to fit with my new slim body. I know it sounds crazy, as all I ever wanted was to lose the excess bulk to fit into society's acceptable norms. I thought that my whole life would magically be 'right' when the weight disappeared.*

Being thin doesn't change your neurological wiring; therefore all your issues don't miraculously disappear. And there's no guarantee that Prince Charming will pass by in his Lamborghini to sweep you into forever-loving arms. Yes, your life will change, but not as you expect. Your relationship with yourself is challenged and your relationships with those around you also shift. It can be disappointing how little spiritual and emotional reward there is in being thin. It can actually be quite a traumatic experience unless you have found your Essential Self and can lean on your own strength.

BEING THIN…
…doesn't mean your life suddenly has purpose and meaning.
Being 1.68m and weighing 115lbs, you'd think that would be it. But keeping that up is hard, hard work. I'd hoped that once I got to my goal weight I

would find contentment. After a while you start having these thoughts of: Is this what life's about?

…doesn't mean your relationships become more functional and that you suddenly have this fabulous social life you've always dreamed of.
When I was in my twenties, I was thin and certainly didn't like myself. My experiences with men were painful to say the least. I was thin but still lonely beyond what I could bear – so most nights I drank myself into a 'coma'.

…doesn't mean you'll be having more fun.
For body fun I belly-dance and have done so for five years. Strangely, as I began to lose weight I stopped dancing in shows. I no longer want to be seen as 'the fat girl'. Yet once, at close to 400lbs, I was shaking my stuff with impunity. Go figure!

…can make you fear yourself.
My mother is known for her extramarital affairs. In my teenage years I had to hear from everybody that I look just like my mother, and that I am just as warm and spontaneous as she is. But I feared becoming like her. When I lost weight I felt fantastic, and loved the compliments from everybody, especially the opposite sex. But then my best friend's husband started to compliment me and was sending me SMS's; I started to feel uncomfortable. With more introspection, I realized I did not trust myself.

…can fill you with fear.
I never believed I'd not be happy to lose weight. I've been noticing my clothes getting loose so I weighed myself to find I have lost 18lbs! I'm in fact worried – scared – that something is wrong, because I'm certainly not dieting. Several of my loved ones (including my dad) experienced weight loss, and were praised to high heaven by the family and others, only to die of cancer shortly afterwards.

…can change the dynamics in your relationships.
For me it's this pushy-husband thing. The minute I lose weight, he starts wanting me to join him in all sorts of activities that I'm not interested in. There is this ever-increasing pressure for me to extend myself and my personality. He's forever pushing me to go further, be more adventurous.

…can make you feel invaded.
When I was fat, the bathroom was my own. Now that I'm thinner, my boyfriend wants to come into my private space and bath me.

...can change your expectations of your partner.
It's like my getting thinner has changed the balance in our relationship. Before we each had a vice: my eating, his drinking, and that maintained some kind of balance. Now that I'm thin, I can't bear his drinking and it's causing arguments galore!

...doesn't mean your relationship with a significant other will improve.
My husband was always comparing me to other women – I was always the fat ugly one. I nearly killed myself to get to my goal weight, but now he just finds other things about me to criticise.

...can cause jealousy to emerge.
My husband is convinced that I'm going to leave him. His jealously since I've lost weight is driving me nuts.

...doesn't mean you'll like your body, or that you'll make peace with all parts of yourself.
I still don't like my body. My legs always appear huge, no matter what I weigh.

...doesn't mean that you feel any better proportioned.
Being pear-shaped, I tend to keep my weight on my thighs and the rest of my body is skinny. So by the time my legs are the way I want them, my face looks tired and my boobs are droopy. And I'm still stuck with the cellulite.

...doesn't mean that you stop comparing yourself to others.
Last year this time I was 62lbs lighter. Looking back, I was thin but I still felt like the ugly duckling.

...doesn't get you out of the vicious cycle.
Once you get there you think the battle is won. Not so because the next battle starts –trying to stay there. I also find once I get to the weight I want to be, I don't stay satisfied with that; it never actually stops. It's an ongoing battle and the question is: Will I ever be satisfied? Because you haven't really dealt with your issues, you have this emptiness inside, like: Why am I not happier?

It can be alarming to realize that you're still not happy when your body is where you've always wanted it to be. This is because we get temporary *pleasure* from external things like appearance and possessions, but lasting *happiness* only comes from an internal source. If you've only changed your exterior, your relationship with life in general won't have changed in any permanent way.

Many Dietonians are blissfully unaware of the pitfalls of being thin because they believe the cultural messages they receive – that thinness automatically equals health, wealth and happiness. We all assume that once we've finally reached Thinland, we'll be able to relax now. This is not so! *I enjoyed the way I looked in the mirror but the maintenance got to me, and the pressure of staying at that weight was taking over my mind and my life. Go to gym; eat only low-fat, low-carb food. And beating yourself up because over the weekend you messed up your whole diet. Striving for perfection has left me in a worse state than before.*

If you still have to restrict and deprive yourself, food remains your enemy. You monitor your eating and use laxatives, appetite suppressants or diuretics to keep your weight at your goal level – you're not *at* goal, you're *in* gaol! Your moods are still reliant on your body looking a particular way. *Feeling good only lasted as long as the scale said what I wanted to see, as long as I could fit into my favorite pants.*

Escaping Diet City is a gradual process in which your mind has to take the lead. While your body is able to change relatively quickly, a mind made of concrete (a rigid, entrenched mindset) can take a lot longer to soften and remould.

You do not need to change your body shape or size or become eternally thin to leave Diet City. You can be overweight and closer to Nature's Valley than a person who is clothes-hanger-thin. **Success doesn't necessarily show up in the size of your body; it shows up in your attitudes and habits, in how comfortable, vibrant and alive you feel living in your body.**

Chapter 5:
♥
Self-love is...

In 2006 I did a series of body-empowerment workshops for a prominent woman's magazine. At the first workshop I looked around alarmed. Sitting around the tables were impeccably made-up, beautiful slim women. What *were* they doing at a body-empowerment workshop? I had my suspicions and I asked, 'How many of you in this room would like to be married to the voice you hear in your head when you look in the mirror?'

Only two hands in the entire hall went up. For the rest of the room, the harsh inner critic within each woman was constantly judging her so that, if verbalised, the voice would be offensive. Think about it: if someone else tells you, 'You're fat and revolting,' you'd be upset and hurt. *So, does saying it to yourself over and over make it okay*? Talk about double standards!

Those women in the room were how I once aspired to look (and how I did look when I was at the height of my body hatred and stuck in Diet City). Like me back then, they were living round the clock with 'someone' (themselves) exacerbating their daily stress by constantly pointing out where they didn't match up. Think of the harm you do to your mental state and your relationships when you self-sabotage like this? As one woman said: *I hated myself so much I was trying to make everyone around me hate me too, and then my self-hatde would be justified.*

But most importantly, what harm does living with this constant internal critic do to our cells, our immune system and ultimately our health? When you're trapped in self-hatred, you'll find that the goal posts are forever moving. *After years of hating myself, I realized that it didn't seem to matter what size I was, there was always a size that seemed better.* That's because self-hatred can never really get you to where you want to be. *Screaming at me, hating myself, restricting myself is not helping. I haven't ever lost weight being like that. What a lot of hating and screaming for nothing!*

Remember, we *always* respond better to love than hate, so what good does being be so mean to yourself do? You know that golden rule: treat others as you'd like to be treated yourself? How about flipping that round and treating *yourself* as you'd really like others to treat you? Being self-loving is living life intelligently. After all those years of dieting and disliking yourself, if it was such a wonderful cure-all, you'd all be living in Nature's Valley by now. Why insist on keeping on doing something that hasn't worked in the past, won't work in the future, and makes you feel more desperate so that you eat more? Do you have anything to lose by choosing self-love over self-dislike? More importantly, what do you gain?

Members of the Mind over Fatter online e.mentoring group (it's free – sign up at www.ditch-diets-live-light.com) continually comment on what a difference is made by the love, kindness and acceptance they experience in the group. Sadly though, most body pilgrims find it vastly easier to be supportive and loving towards others than towards themselves. I can't say this strongly enough: *It is never more beneficial to be self-hating than self-loving.*

Many body pilgrims will struggle with this idea of self-love. We've always been told that self-love is selfish (not!), arrogant (not that either) and indulgent (nor this). We often feel we have to hide those wonderful parts of ourselves to prevent us from being considered conceited or vain. So we hardly dare to love ourselves in healthy and respecting ways. But loving yourself not only enriches your life, but also the lives of those around you when they interact with the fulfilled, happy person you become. Consider that you've been created in your Creator's image (and by 'Creator' I mean whatever God-figure you feel comfortable with, be that God, Allah, Buddha, Krishna, the Universe, the Source or any other.) You have all been imbued with Creator-like qualities – which are not about achieving a certain 'perfect' weight or fitting into a particular size of clothing. Nowhere in any holy text have I found any references that dictate what physical measurements our Creator expects us to conform to! Creator-like qualities consist of values such as patience, compassion, love, tolerance and acceptance. These are what we should be encouraged to cultivate.

If you're still struggling with applying those Creator-like qualities to yourself, think of the religious tenet, Love your neighbour as yourself. This implies that you need to have self-love that at the least is equal to the love you might have for others.

Do you remember those old 'Love is…' cartoons by Kim featuring the two nude innocents? Well the Nature's Valley cartoon strip features a 'Self-love is…' series. Its central theme is returning to a state of innocence, to a time before cultural beliefs about our body become engraved into our neural pathways.

Be warned though, self-loving actions on the The Joy-Filled Body journey are often exactly opposite to the ones you're used to. In Diet City it is good to weigh yourself; in Nature's Valley that can be a particularly non-self-loving act. [31] *I made the mistake of weighing myself at gym the other night. It's so depressing. Guess how I handled the extreme stress of my weight gain? Malva pudding and cream, of course! The scale is an evil invention.* Diet City tells you having lists of illegal and legal foods is a way of taking care of yourself. In Nature's Valley self-love is making all foods 'legal'. *I just wanted to say that I've definitely made progress in my journey. I still eat junk, but I no longer feel ashamed and I no longer beat myself up.* By Diet City standards this would not be progress. It would evoke a howling protest of, 'If you're eating junk food *and* not feeling guilty, you're going backwards, not forwards. You're letting yourself go!' Diet City encourages you to punish yourself with guilt when you don't stick to a diet.

In Nature's Valley dieting and guilt destroy self-love. Diet City wants you to compare yourself with others. In Nature's Valley, the belief is that comparisons are often the swiftest route to destroying self-love. *Every page I turned there were more beautiful bodies to see – I felt sick when I realized how far I was from ever matching that. How do they get to be so cellulite free?* Self-loving actions include trusting your body and being gentle with yourself when you forget to live in body-wise ways. So let's meander down the self-love labyrinth into Nature's Valley.

SELF-LOVE IS KNOWING THIS JOURNEY IS A SPIRITUAL ONE

Self ♥ = remembering that self-love is our birthright

Why are we so drawn to babies? Because of their innocence. They remind us of how we were before we forgot we were sacred, of what we can return to become – beings with unlimited possibilities. As toddlers we lived in our bodies in a carefree state. We were still living in Nature's Valley; we hadn't yet forgotten our sacredness by becoming preoccupied with the outer illusions proffered as steps to happiness. Indeed, the belief that we can never be thin or rich enough go way beyond the logical. *If a genie had to pop out of a magic lamp and grant me three wishes, one would be to be thin. Somehow deep down in my psyche – much deeper than my logic can reach – is still the thought that if I was thin (and wealthy), then my life would be better. I would be accepted into the 'in' crowd, and I'd be able to afford doing what I wanted in life. If I was thin I'd automatically get everyone's approval and admiration, not their scorn and disdain.*

We need to return to that place that existed before our culture infused us with ideas of what we need to do (and become) in order to get ahead. That place where we recognise that self-love and self-esteem are our birthright. *I always think – how can we possibly expect to 'hear' our own body's signals of hunger, fullness, sadness, accurately if we don't value our body's worth?! In other words, we cannot ever hope to break free from the chains of emotional eating until we can restore (and maintain) our self-esteem.*

Self ♥= realizing we are much more than our physical body

A major key to escaping Diet City is when we really 'get it' that the physical is only one aspect of our bodies. *The one thing that really worked for me in terms of being able to honour myself by no longer abusing myself with food was to have a concrete body cast done. It is a cast of my torso (at my maximum) and the day I looked at it – really studied it – and admitted to myself that the cast was really quite beautiful, like an ancient fertility goddess, was the day that I was able to relinquish the constant need to feed in an uncontrolled and frenzied manner. It is hanging on the wall in my TV room as a constant reminder that my body is (was) beautiful! Another aid has been hot rock massage. I go to an alternative therapist and the physical, emotional and spiritual nurturing that's part of each session has been invaluable to me.* Leaving behind the identity of a Dietonian is multi-pronged – it's a physical, emotional and spiritual liberation. Just tackling your eating or your exercising isn't enough – this really does need to be a holistic approach if we're to find lasing peace.

Self ♥= realizing that self-acceptance is found *within*

Advertisers would have us believe that the answer to every problem exists in bottles on shelves; that the solution is an easy matter of 'swallow this pill,' 'drink this potion' or 'rub on this lotion'. What these don't do is teach you self-acceptance. *My problem? Self-acceptance! Can't one buy it in a bottle somewhere? Previously I thought it was hidden in all the diet potions and pills, but at the end I realized it was not. You see, if I want something, I want it now – instant gratification! Now I know that self-acceptance has to come from within me. But it is taking so long...* Being mean to yourself isn't going to get you anywhere healthy. *I'm the one step forward, two steps back pilgrim. Beating me up about it is not going to make the unwanted, extra me disappear. So it is back to Square One again. Time for some tender loving care for myself.* Try to take yourself back to the days as a very young child when you had no interest in potions or lotions, and your happiness didn't originate from your looks, products or possessions, it just bubbled out from within.

Self ♥=believing in yourself

Western cultural beliefs have taken our thinking and whisked it down the rabbit hole, where it's been turned upside down, inside out and twirled around so we're facing the wrong way – focusing on the exterior. Having myself obsessively exercised down to a teeny 92lbs, I imagined I'd feel like an absolute princess. But those external changes weren't enough to fill me with confidence or wipe out my bad body thoughts. It really is all about how *you* are seeing yourself in your head.

When I was in my early twenties I probably weighed 175-195lbs. I refused to date, because I thought my body was disgusting – how could any man find me attractive? Then in my mid-twenties I weighed 265–285lbs – but I felt attractive and had a lot more male attention than when I weighed 195lbs! It's all about the confidence. And, until that confidence comes naturally, I say, 'Fake it till you make it'. If you're thinking, I'm not going to lie to myself, pretending I'm the confident person I'm not, consider this: you're already lying if you tell yourself you aren't worthy of love. So, if you're going to 'lie' to yourself at least choose a 'lie' that has a base of truth – fake that self-love until it finds its way back to you.

I was experiencing the agony of self-loathing, and dreading going to a party, when my aunt took me aside. She told me that if I went into that hall feeling like a queen, walking like a queen, showing the whole world how self-confident and self-assured I was, I would actually start feeling like a queen and lose my shyness. I must be a wonderful actress, because within TEN MINUTES I already had two guys dancing with me. I spent the whole evening (including Mills & Boon-style romantic walks on the beach later) with one of them! Acting 'as if' is extremely powerful because you get out of your ego's way long enough to allow your Essential Self to surface again.

SELF-LOVE IS OUTSTING OUTDATED HABITS

Self ♥= debunking cultural myths

The deep essential truths (you are all born equal and special) are enduring and empowering and don't change historically, or from one culture to another. Surface ego beliefs (the shape of your body is what makes you special) are never stable; they're the ones that create self-doubt. Challenging surface beliefs is absolutely central to escaping Diet City. Fortunately, a bit of further investigation easily debunks the myths. *Instead of lusting after the glamorous lifestyles of pop divas and movie stars, I've started watching out for stories about their lives. What I've discovered is that, despite being physically beautiful and unbelievably wealthy, they live crazy, unhappy lives. I no longer believe that when I'm gorgeous, the world will be my oyster. I've taken a lot of pressure off myself to become something I never can.*

You already are all that you ever need to be, and you don't need to become 'anything' or 'anybody'. Look for those misleading contradictions in Western society's false belief systems. *Why is it that with the first skinny swimwear-model you see, you're already comparing your body to hers when in reality you go to the mall and to the beach and you see only one in a million?* Ask yourself instead, how do your apparent imperfections create wonderful aspects of your body? *I realized I didn't actually want to be model-like. My imperfect body had shaped parts of me I really liked. It helped me conform less, which strengthened me. It also gave me a rather quirky sense of humour about myself.*

Looking back at the bodies from other eras very clearly illustrates why today's standards of beauty aren't deep truths. *I've been drawing people inside my head, using the poses from a book of erotic photos circa 1920. They are photos of real women and yet they're so beautiful. What was shocking was that I realized these would never get published today. They look nothing like the bits of jerky featured in today's magazines. It's made me feel quite different about my body.*

Self ♥= refusing to compare yourself unfavorably

Our modern culture teaches us to become comparison-based. *It's that feeling of, by most other people's standards they've got it made – and I clearly haven't.* Again, remember that everyone was created equal – and not terms of looks, possessions or achievements. Only your ego-self makes comparisons. Comparisons are bred out of feelings of being separate. You see others as competitors against which to measure yourself. The following Dietonian 'had it all' yet still concludes: *I still sat at my daughter's ballet lessons on my own, wanting so badly to fit in with the other mothers who I felt were looking at me up and down ... I STILL felt inferior to them!* 'Having it all' on the exterior doesn't take away inferior feelings on the interior. Ego-imposed standards become an ever-moving target. Until you grow in self-love, any changes you make to your body don't touch you where it counts – in your heart. As one Dietonian escapee pointed out: *If our full value as human beings is what's on top of our skin (that's less than skin deep!), it's no wonder we feel tense almost all the time.* That constant tense state is far more health-eroding than carrying your few extra kilos. When we're constantly casing our eyes sideways to compare ourselves we're flooding our biochemistry and changing how our bodies function.

Self ♥= not buying into beliefs that promote body-obsession

Self-love is doing things that reduce your body obsessions – and that's not setting yourself an unreachable goal that prepares you for certain failure because it was a ridiculous goal in the first place. *For a while I was so obsessed with those fitness girls, my biggest wish was to be like that. I bought the magazines and subscribed to a newsletter. I tried to buy all the equipment, as well as the supplements. Needless to say, I never got near that dream. And the more unreachable it looked the more I criticised myself for not having the willpower and discipline to become like that.*

What we think of as a successful goal needs a radical overhaul. Ms Fitness is about obsessively limiting your life and your love of it too – it's not about attaining self-love. *Obsession is not a word, it's a lifestyle! You live, eat, sleep and urinate Ms Fitness, it totally consumes your life. Compulsive is not a lifestyle, it's a rule! Everything about gaining fitness is compulsive from the food to the training to the competitions, and worst of all your physical appearance! Some of the competitors even sold their houses to support their habit! My family started telling me I'd become cold and judgemental of others. I was so lonely, my friends couldn't put up with me talking about Ms Fitness ALL the time.* Self-love is not about doing obsessive exercise that's harmful to your body, feeling superior to others, becoming judgemental of people or becoming isolated. Self-love is when your Essential Self shouts at you and you *listen.*

So you're probably asking yourself, what made me stop? Well here it is: After my first competition my coaches said the only way to first or second place was to start taking steroids! I had already had a boob job; now drugs, what next? Nooo, thank you!

Self ♥= no longer giving your 'imperfections' airtime

It's simply not helpful or self-loving to keep zoning in on parts of your self you don't like. Nor is it to continually point those parts out to others. Why keep alive your hurt when there are so many other things to talk about and turn your mind to? *Since I've started being more accepting of my body and its imperfections, I've noticed that I have different conversations with people. I'm no longer constantly pointing out where I don't match up and since I've stopped doing this, I've noticed other people have also stopped commenting on my body.*

Okay, so some of you are still very dubious about this whole idea of self-love. It's difficult to change beliefs that have been held for so many years, and which fly in the face of popular opinion – a bit like one tiny fish trying to swim against the shoal. As one Mind over Fatter pilgrim put it:

It's tough to be the small minority that pushes against the grain of the media and society. It's tough to feel like we 'don't fit in' to the accepted 'norm'. But I'm starting to think that our Maker knows that, and has specially made us big enough to stand up to them and join hands to unite!

Self ♥= reframing things for ourselves

Dietonians usually pass the unkindest comments on their various body parts – they benefit from finding kinder ways of talking about themselves. Many women hate their 'hams' – their upper arms. A conversation about big arms amongst the online group led to this adaptation of *Little Red Riding Hood*: *Little Red Riding Hood (looking at grandma): 'Ooh, Grandma, what big arms you have!' Grandma: 'All the better to hug you with!'* Of course, arms aren't the only cause of anxiety for Dietonians. *Both my gran and mother have big thighs, so mine are genetic. But no amount of hating my thighs was going to improve matters. So I started treating them as if I loved them because of the link they gave me with my grandmother, who was now dead (but whose big lap I'd loved to sit on). That helped enormously. Instead of seeing them as hated parts of myself, I saw them as comforting parts of my grandmother. It also helped me to remember that I hadn't loved her any less because she had big thighs – nor, in fact, had I ever really noticed them until my own thighs became a problem!*

We are prone to thinking that the parts of our bodies we dislike so much are all that others notice about us. It is so far from the truth. *Whenever I think people are noticing my fat butt, I remind myself that they are too busy noticing the parts of themselves they dislike to worry about me. Besides, if my butt worries them, it's their problem, not mine.*

Self ♥= seeing ourselves through different eyes

Witnessing how we *don't* want our lives to be can be an important catalyst. *Watching my sister nearly kill herself just to be thin, made me decide that being thin is not everything. She drank 10 mugs of coffee a day, ate about nothing and ran three times per day for between 45 minutes and 1 hour a time. I barely saw her as she was too afraid to gain an ounce. I decided that I do not want to go that way, and stopped all my diets. Now I constantly tell myself to accept the way I look and that 'my body and mind are under construction'.* Sometimes witnessing ourselves through others also helps us realize we are stuck in thinking that belongs in another generation. Says a 40-plus body pilgrim:

I was reading a letter from a 22-year-old describing her imaginary universe in which she one day weighed a specific figure. It made me realize I was somehow still stuck in that 22-year-old mindset when I no longer had to be.

Looking through old photographs or other memorabilia can jolt us into seeing now what we couldn't see then. *As a teen I hated myself so much that I used to cut myself out of every picture. But not so long ago, my sister had all our ancient family videos put onto DVD and for the first time I could see myself at that age again. Well, I was absolutely amazed to watch myself as the 16-year-old that I had so hated. I was in a bikini and had a really great body (in terms of Western standards), and I was actually quite stunning. Yes, really, I was! So, if what I saw then was a revolting me, I can take what I see now a lot less seriously. It helped me see that how I view myself is incredibly distorted.*

Self ♥= noticing what you normally wouldn't

I remember my own Dietonian days. Somehow my focus never extended beyond seeing what I *didn't* have. It only saw beautiful bodies and filtered out the rest – but liberation from Diet City requires a different focus. *The pool area was filled with beautiful bodies... so I tried to do something totally new. Instead of comparing myself to the beautiful bodies, I tried to see the bodies that were not 'perfect'. And you know what – I saw LOTS of them! They were all shapes and sizes; many were even bigger than me! Suddenly I didn't feel so self-conscious any more. I swam for the first time in ages in my bathing costume rather than those horrible baggy shorts to cover up my thighs, and I had a fantastic time doing it. I realized we all have different shapes, and we're all okay.*

SELF-LOVE IS RIDDING YOURSELF OF DIET CITY

Self ♥= having a sense of humour

When you learn to lighten up and take this whole body thing a lot less seriously, you can laugh at situations that once had the potential to make you cry and gnash your teeth; you can let them bother you a whole lot less. *Trying on swimming costumes is one of life's trials. One flattened my breasts as if they were cookies on a baking sheet while the rest of me oozed out like raw dough. I tried tiger stripes, but Victoria's Secret isn't ready for me yet! As for*

101

the black number, it looked like a black cushion on a lumpy pink sofa. What can a girl say – I can either hate myself or have a sense of humour! Either way, I'll still be fat. The question is do I want to fill my fat with hate or with humour? This body pilgrim has got one thing right. Hate is a low-energy attractor pattern that destroys those beautiful shape-forming crystals in your cells (remember Dr Emoto Masaru?) and ultimately affects your health negatively.

Self ♥= freeing yourself from Diet City paraphernalia

Personally, I love the cartoon of the woman lying on her back with her scale balanced on her feet in the air. Now, that's a self-loving way to use them! I think scales definitely suit fish more than they do women. Then again, aren't we a little like fish? A fish doesn't know it's wet and in water; we don't know just how immersed we are in Diet City beliefs. We may not have scales covering our bodies, but we have scales dictating the quality of our lives. Where fish scales give the fish its beauty, we use the scales in our lives to achieve a distorted sense of beauty. But no more!

Its self-love to get rid of all the stuff that has kept you trapped in the diet cycle. *I threw out my huge pile of diet magazines. I used to buy every single diet/shape/fitness magazine – anything with the word 'diet' on the cover – then keep them just in case I needed to refer back to their 'wisdom!'* Or at least to realize how unhelpful the stuff is and resolve no longer to use it. *I think that some of my pants feel looser these days, but I am not going to step on that scale! I know that stupid piece of equipment still has such a lot of power over me. Let's just say I still have a tendency towards numberitis.*

Self ♥= letting go of Diet City fat-judgements

In 1999, I bought Marilynn Wann's book Fat! So? And after reading it I actually became okay with calling myself fat, because I realized fat isn't bad or good, it just is. Why should I be hurt when someone calls me fat? I'm not hurt when someone calls me female or tells me I have medium length hair. Try to see 'fat' as just a word. It's only our culture that fills the word with such negative connotations. When you learn how to quieten the voice of judgement that has taken a word and attached to it connotations of laziness, being weak-willed, a no-good slob, you go a long way towards not harming your health or your self-esteem (remember Emoto's shattered water crystals when exposed to derogatory phrases?). Doing anything that prevents harm to your health or confidence is a self-loving action.

Self ♥= having 'under reconstruction' mentality

If you've managed to diet yourself fatter and are now starting your journey of liberation from Diet City, it's far more helpful to think of your life and body (note: I didn't only say 'body') as being in various stages of remodelling. *A year ago I weighed 55lbs less than today. It's not easy when I get in front of my cupboard and have nothing to wear. I don't even want to go to church because I just know what the people will think (they never knew about the fad diets, pills and potions). I can't tell you the shame I feel every time I go out in public. I wish I could wear a sign around my neck saying 'Body and soul under Mind over Fatter construction'.* Where you are *now* is what's important. Reconstruction does not happen instantly – think of renovating a building. You need to take it step by step, day by day.

SELF-LOVE IS REALIZING RELATIONSHIPS HAVE TO CHANGE
(including the one you have with yourself)

Self ♥= acknowledging everyone has a reason for being in your life

Even those who evoke strong negative emotions in your life are your 'teachers' in one or other way, whether the person is a caring mother or gentle sibling – or an irritating partner, vexing friend or critical in-law. *My mother-in-law is so critical of everyone's bodies. It makes me feel really vulnerable. But it helps to remind me that sometimes people are there to teach us how we don't want to be.*

Learn what you can from these individuals, both how you want and don't want to be. But also be prepared to recognise when someone's role in your life has become redundant. Be grateful for whatever lessons they helped you learn, then let them go emotionally – not because you judge yourself as better than them but because you want to create space for new teachers. *Some friends have fallen by the wayside as I've come to realize that I was the comfort in their lives – the 'fat' one who allowed them to feel superior or the 'fatter' one so they didn't appear so big.*

Self ♥= accepting changing relationships

When you grow, relationships with significant others will change. *We've had a good many rough patches as my weight seemed to overshadow the family. My husband has had to learn that I will no longer accept being treated with less care and courtesy than he gives to a stranger. My children now have a mom who can do more with them as well as around the house; I'm more fun to be with.* Such changes will not always be welcomed. *I feel that the new me has been trying to do what is the right thing for me, rather than what people would want me to do and I have seen results. But I discovered this week that my hubby is still feeling very threatened by the changed me. He feels that he's the only one that is 'bearing the brunt' of my new ways and that I have become a more selfish person.* Sticking to the changed you in the face of opposition can be one of the most self-loving things you do in the long term.

Self ♥= doing what's difficult

Be aware that it's going to be difficult to change ingrained habits, but it will be worth it because to escape Diet City permanently, it's not your body where the greatest changes have to happen. *For the first time I was really honest and did not 'sugarcoat' anything. It was exhausting because I brought quite a few issues to the table. Once one was resolved, the next was put on the table (note the food connotations). It was no easy road. I first had to get my hubby to sit and listen; I started with the small issues and progressed to the deep-rooted ones. Some of the things he told me about myself were true and hard to 'swallow', but they gave me insight into myself.*

It's also about you realizing that you've often created an illusion about how your life was.

I think that men, in particular, feel threatened by change – my hubby has known me a certain way for 30 years! Our entire marriage was based on my 'old' ways of falling over me to please everyone; now suddenly he has to get used to my totally different ways. It goes to show how hard we worked to keep things smooth – at our own expense. But was that just the illusion we wanted to give everyone else? My marriage was very rocky and I had severe food obsessions. Personally, I was in such a deep depressive state that I was almost suicidal at times. It's just so tempting sometimes to go back to when everything went smoothly! I know now that all the things I experienced were pieces of my journey and that I had to go through them learn about me. That's the wonderful thing about this journey – it's sometimes difficult to keep going, but you can never turn back.

Self ♥= protecting yourself

Self-love is standing up for your new personal boundaries. *I went to the doctor yesterday because I was suffering from back pains. I told him I was aware my weight could be playing some role, but that I was treating my eating disorder and was not allowed to diet.*

Self ♥= choosing positive forces in your life

Looking at yourself through the eyes of someone who has confidence in you can remind you of the forgotten parts of your Essential Self. Seek out the company of people who believe in you because they will enable you to crawl out from under your social conditioning and view yourself through their eyes. *Having one person believe in you can make the difference. It can act as a catalyst.*

Self ♥= making 'you' choices even when others press you to make 'their' choices

Everyone else seems to have ideas about the body you should have. Wouldn't it be a self-loving action to rely on your own body to dictate the size it wants to be? *Why do I have to be a size 10, 12 or even 14, when I don't know what my natural size will be once I start living the life I truly want to live? Once I start listening to my body, well, who knows...? I might end up an athletic size 12.* Through a lack of understanding, not all the choices you make during your escape from Diet City will sit comfortably with others. *When I first started my journey my hubby had no idea of what I was trying to do, especially when I started to stock up with formerly illegal foods. His anger against me was not badly intended – he was just very scared that here I was, off on some hare-brained scheme to hurt myself once again!*

SELF-LOVE IS ACTING WITH A LONG TERM VIEWPOINT

Self ♥= making baby steps towards being more self-loving

For some pilgrims, leaping from self-hating to self-loving thoughts and actions is simply too great a jump. So, be self-loving by recognizing and placing smaller stepping stones in-between. *I can still connect with respecting myself enough – but loving myself like that... it's still 'pie in the sky' stuff for me.*

Moving back to being self-loving seldom happens in an instant unless you're having one of the paradigm-shifting aha moments that occur from time to time. When these happen, it's usually because you're suddenly able to see another viewpoint. Usually, progress is slow – first stopping the harsh criticism, then starting to reframe your idea of yourself, next starting to respect yourself, accepting yourself, and so on. *Some days are easier than others when it comes to loving myself.*

Self ♥= abandoning constantly trying harder

Sometimes the harder you try; the more elusive it becomes to get where you want to go. Then giving up the struggle can be the most self-loving action to take. *My mother has been a compulsive overeater and bulimia sufferer for as long as I can remember. Growing up I watched her going to individual and group therapy, I watched with dread as she climbed on the scale to see if it would be a 'good' or a 'bad' day. Diet books lined our bookshelves and I saw how limiting it was. I was so fearful I'd grow up to be like her. It became a self-fulfilling prophecy. Whether I was thin or fat, it made no difference – my weight still ruled my life. I got to a point where I was so sick of the constant effort that I was able to escape from my mother's shadow. Key was that I finally gave up trying so hard, and it was effortless. I ate whatever I wanted, whether it was Kentucky Fried Chicken or salad. When I let go of obsessing about food, it was as if it finally let go of me. Sometimes we don't have to try harder, we have to try less!*

Self ♥= making self-loving choices for the long term

You may well ask why I place so much emphasis on making those self-loving choices. Personally, when I love or am 'in like' with myself, I find it much easier to make choices that allow my body to settle at its natural size. Not the cultural or insurance ideal, but the size that's naturally right for it. *If I truly loved it, I would want to take care of it and nurture it with whatever is best for it.*

Being duped by a thin-obsessed culture into thinking you don't have the right to love yourself when your body doesn't match current cultural depictions is being deceitful to yourself. You're worthy and fabulous right now! *We practice self-deceit. We choose things that are bad for us and convince ourselves we like them, or need them (or they need us). A good thing would have been to learn to like myself more. Good things build me as a person, for example, finding a God inside that loves me; nature; affirming, kind, loving people; creative expression. Bad things take away from me, make me feel bad about myself – for example, a person who breaks me down or who wants me to be something I'm not. Using something to make me forget is not a good thing. I use sugar, lying to myself that it will make me feel better. Actually, it makes me feel worse because it keeps me fat. Instead of doing things I love, I stay at home and eat sweet things till my tummy's full. Then I don't feel like doing anything or seeing anyone.* Analyze what are good and bad choices for you. Ask yourself if you'd find it easier to make good choices if you were self-loving or self-hating.

SELF-LOVE IS NOT WAITING TO LIVE LIFE

Self ♥ = not letting Diet City hooks put you on hold

Be it a wedding, a school reunion or any other celebratory occasion, it's all too common for this kind of event to lure you back into your Diet City cycle. *I have been thinking of going on an emergency diet since Friday as we've decided to go to Austria after Christmas. All I can think about is that I'm not fitting into my skinny jeans and I don't want to go on holiday if I can't look and feel great! But the more I think about dieting and losing those dreaded kg's the more I want to eat until I OD on sugar.* DON'T DO IT! Because, as the above morsel indicates, just the thought of starting your cycle of deprivation once more is enough to start you eating all over again. It only takes a sniff of restriction to send us back. It's as if there's a silent part of us that recognizes we cannot be suppressed in this way and rebels.

Self ♥ = living a full life NOW

Most inhabitants of Diet City are waiting until they have the 'right' body to begin living the life they want to live – but, in fact, you deserve to have what you want *now*. Being thin doesn't suddenly make you worthy of the job you'd like or meaningful relationships or wearing clothes you find attractive. Making the decision that you are worthy makes your life worthy – and ready to be lived in full *now. One thing that helped me was this visualisation from Overcoming Overeating by Hirschmann and Munter. They tell you to imagine that a strange wind blows over the world, and putting us into a state where our weight will never, ever change – despite what we eat or don't eat. How would you live your life if you knew with absolute certainty that how you are now is what you will look like for the rest of your life? The visualisation helped me start to accept my natural body shape with a bit more compassion. It also helps push away those hateful thoughts.* If you're trapped in Diet City, just the thought of this visualisation is paralysing – but think of it, just on the other side of paralysis lies freedom. What if, instead of waiting until you reached some aspired-for figure on a scale, you started living now? What would you do differently? In what ways would you stop limiting yourself? It could be quite exhilarating. Apply the energy you were spending on dieting to living fully. *If I think back to all the weight I've lost and regained . . . what a waste of my time. I just think of all the living I've missed out on while obsessing about food!*

Self ♥= indulging in letting self-love in

Participate in life, go out with friends, show up at social occasions – don't miss out on all the fun. *I have become less isolated. I went out with friends twice in the last ten days. I realized I was staying home, waiting until I got thin to go out.*

Buy yourself attractive clothes that fit well and look good on your shape *now. I went and bought nice comfortable clothes that fitted me as I am at the moment, not two sizes too small like I did when I refused to buy anything bigger than my desired size. Just by allowing the slightly overweight me to wear something pretty in a size that's quite normal and acceptable have made me feel more self-loving!*

Pick up the courage to take a big step towards you having more fun. *It's a breakthrough for me to go to this ball! I refuse to put my life on hold anymore. I'm choosing to dance, choosing to live. I have this feeling of; once I take these courageous steps, things will fall into place. I feel like God is trying to tell me, 'I will orchestrate to make things happen for you.' Ooh wee, life is good! Life is for the living and I choose to live!*

Take the step to look out for your health *today. I've been feeling this pain for THREE years, all the while blaming myself, blaming my weight but desperately waiting to lose some kilograms before going to the doctor. Isn't it crazy to suffer for three years because you're waiting to get thin?*

SELF-LOVE IS BEING KIND TO YOURSELF

Self ♥= giving yourself the leeway you give others

Time and time again, I see Dietonians treating themselves in ways they would never treat another person. I also see how supportive and accepting they are of others who are self-hating. *I am my own worst enemy, my worst judge. When I 'see' myself through the eyes of others, it's only to discover that they are not nearly as judgemental as I am.* The average Dietonian needs to recognise her double standards. For example, she would never reject another person for the things she rejects in herself.

Think about your own loved ones. Would you love your husband any less if he had a big tummy? Or a bald head? Or he was disfigured with a scar on his face? Would you say, 'Darling, I don't love you anymore because you're not perfect?' Then why would you say these things to yourself? Isn't it ironic that we fall so easily in love with other people but we find it so difficult to love ourselves? Self-love is in fact the best form of love!

Self ♥= being accepting – and curious

Think about the options you have when you observe your body going through its natural changes. You could accept them, or at the very least sit back and watch with curiosity, or you could get frantic and feel fearful. I recently shared this with the Mind over Fatter e-mentoring group. *After years of being pretty much at one weight and fitting into the same jeans I did 10–12 years ago while having no less body fun, I suddenly experienced a fat-spurt. I watched with great curiosity. What was my body trying to tell me? I noticed my menstrual cycle was changing, I had hot flushes and night sweats, and I was growing a walrus moustache and chin hairs (made only more prolific by my attempts at waxing because some advertisement had conned me into increasing them so I'd need their product more.) So I decided to sit back and watch what unfolds with interest because my body is doing what it needs to at this stage of my life.* What happened was that I felt calm instead of frantic. This also prevented me from being lured back into Diet City. Gaining the weight isn't a disaster. It's simply a message from my body. My self-loving action is to decipher what my body is trying to tell me, and decide calmly how to go from there.

Finally, if you treat yourself and your body only with respect and care, you will eventually get there. *I no longer beat myself up when I make unwise decisions. If I do something stupid, I acknowledge that it was stupid, then I let it go. I don't spend hours stewing over it, telling myself I'm stupid and a failure. Instead I tell myself that I'll just keep on trying. Get up and keep walking.*

Chapter 6:

♥

Body-play

As children we were very active, had a low percentage of body fat and used calories as fast as we consumed them. But as we grew up and became more 'sensible,' we slowly also become more sedentary. Instead of running, jumping and hopping, we mostly sit and drive so that our muscles are replaced by fat. There is absolutely no doubt that we need to rediscover our childhood joy of 'exercise'.

Having said that, I, like many others, HATE the word exercise! And the reason has nothing to do with hating exercise itself. It has to do with the image and social connotations that have become attached to exercise: 'blood, sweat and tears,' 'no pain, no gain' and 'giving it your all.' It doesn't take much to see the picture: a zealous sergeant-majorish type up front yelling, 'C'mon, step it up, step it up! Faster, faster, lift those knees up, up... Feel the burrrnn!' And fully kitted out in matching Lycra and high-end fashion labels, the steppers comply.

Okay, so you might be thinking, what's so wrong with that? Firstly, there's a sense of needing to do it right and looking sideways as you compare yourself to those around you. Am I kicking high enough? Is my face the only one that's puce? Does anyone *else* look less than perfect in Lycra? Secondly, anything less than feeling the burrrnn and you're supposedly 'being lazy; you may as well not be wasting your time'. *I'd like to start exercising again because I am feeling uncomfortable and stiff, but I just associate it so much with punishment. The only time I've enjoyed it is when it was just a gossipy walk with friends. But then I was told that wasn't aerobic exercise.* Nonsense! Every bit of movement makes a difference (did you know that a wriggler can burn up to 700 calories a day?) – not just the aerobic-related parts. Watch young children – do they obsess about whether its aerobic exercise they're doing? Walking and talking with a friend has great health benefits and is vastly is better than not walking at all.

What's wrong is that we were born loving to be active, but after a lifetime of conditioning in our homes and schools when we were too active and we got into trouble for it, most Dietonians now loathe it. We have psychological hooks about exercise – these are the subconscious snares of your mind that keep you hooked into old attitudes and habits. So you struggle along, from one lapsed exercise contract to another, only strengthening your dislike of anything active so it becomes even more difficult to sustain a healthily active lifestyle. As toddlers and children, our environment was our natural gym and we used it 'spontaneously' (a high-energy attractor pattern), running, jumping, hopping, skipping and climbing at every opportunity. We were seldom still because we didn't know how to be, it wasn't natural to be sedentary. It was natural (a positive-energy attractor pattern) to be active and on the move. *I had a crazy 'dance session' with my kids. They laughed their heads off ... now they keep asking for more.*

The problem with sterile exercise environments is that they have a sense of 'forcedness' (a low-energy attractor pattern). What you do there is usually dictated by someone not living in your body. But get this… once upon a childhood, body-play used to be self-directed fun! We were so unaware of there being a right or a wrong way to moving, or whether we were wearing the 'right' clothes or whether we looked good doing it or not. Watch the glazed faces of the average aerobic zombie pumping it out. Do they look like they're having fun? Do you hear peals of excited laughter? No, fitness is s-e-r-i-o-u-s business! Instead, there's a sense of 'grinning and bearing it', doing this because you *have* to, if you don't then you'll blow up like a balloon. There's a sense of pride in surviving a class in which the instructor 'killed' you– as if getting through such a strenuous class somehow makes you a more superior human being. For some, exercising your way to fitness is a 'sobering' experience (a negative-attractor pattern that weakens your muscle response). Alternatively, joy and humour calibrate above 200, making tested muscles give a strong response. We need to be joyfully about active.

It reminds me of the moment when I hand out balloons in my The Joy-Filled Body workshops – you can sense a new buzz of excitement; the energy in the room is heightened, tangibly. You can *feel* it! Before you know it, adults are dashing around, whooping with childlike wonder and glee, way too engrossed in their game to notice they're running around like a bunch of crazy lunatics. For those few moments, it's as if they're able to step back in time, unearth their childlike spirit and forget themselves in the joy of unrestricted play.   This is something I find the most telling. In the hundreds of workshops I've run, when I've asked, 'How many of you noticed the parts of your body you're normally painfully aware of, and would normally be preoccupied with if you were exercising?' I've never yet had anyone put up their hand. They are so busy 'being' they've had no time to notice what their bodies are doing, like breasts jiggling too much or legs hurting! It's all about giggling and doubling over with breathless laughter. For those few moments, they forget that they hate running around or doing anything that raises a sweat, all because they're back in touch with their fun-filled childlike spirit.

What's wrong with the exercise picture is that we have to sign up for classes to do what we once did naturally as children. And for most people it isn't fun, its torture! That doesn't mean that exercise clubs are bad. But even when I, as a regular gym bunny, showed up regularly every morning at 5:30 come rain, hail or shine, aerobic classes never left me with the same sense of delight and wonder as cartwheels in the back garden did. As Dr Hawkins, whose Map of Consciousness gives us the high- or low-energy attractor patterns, points out, the word 'regulated' calibrates at less than 200 and makes muscles test weak whereas 'free' is a powerful (positive) pattern that makes them test strong. This doesn't mean that regulated exercise doesn't burn up fat and create muscle. It does mean that even the Incredible Hulk's muscles will test weak when responding to 'regulated' and strong in response to 'free'.

So you can eat well, not smoke, not drink and generally live healthily, but without movement, laughter and fun you will never feel as energetic and vibrant as you do when body-*play* is a part of your life. *I make a point of playing games outside with my kids, especially on those long summer evenings. We play hide 'n' seek, hopscotch, let Rover come over, and all those old favorites (we've even done some skipping – remember salt, mustard, vinegar and pepper?). Do you know how wonderful it feels to be tired from playing?*

As Leonardo Buscaglia points out in *Bus 69 to Paradise*, playfulness amongst all forms of life is instinctive and universal. Dolphins, chimpanzees, dogs, cats, squirrels all play; merely watching them splash, chase, and engage in rough and tumble makes you feel more joyful. So why do 'wise' and 'intelligent' humans stop as they get older? From the 'important' grown-ups at home and school we got messages that play wasn't as valuable as work. They encouraged us to give up our 'childish ways', to become serious and engage in mature and productive behaviour. Work got you ahead, playing and dreaming got you nowhere. Anything too raucous or too active got you into trouble or onto medication. We learned that when grown people play, they are 'childish'. But in fact play has multiple benefits. Active play is fabulous for fitness, health and wellbeing.

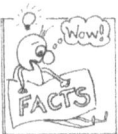

Personal fitness is important. In 1999 Steven N Blair, director of research at the Cooper Institute for Aerobics Research (USA), reported that it was fitness and not the degree of fatness that had the most impact on death rates. Over an eight-year period, fit men – whether lean, normal or obese – had a similar death rate. According to the study, 'Lean men…had increased longevity *only* if they were physically fit; obese men who were fit did not have elevated mortality.'

When you're active, regardless of whether you lose weight or not, there are fabulous health benefits. When the only time that we're doing exercising (and usually hating every moment of it at the same time), because it's a way to lose weight – we're robbing it of something fabulous because it becomes another 'hafta'.

I comment in the Mind over Fatter program manual: 'I find it interesting to note that when people start the Mind over Fatter journey, what they want most is something to tell them exactly what to eat and how much of it. If having what you could eat dictated to you worked so well, I wouldn't be writing this book. The nutritional value of what you put into your mouth is really important for your health as well as to balance your brain chemistry. *But if you want to feel energetic, possibly lose weight healthily and stand a chance of keeping it off – exercise is absolutely one of your most essential allies.'*

So here's the million-dollar question. If you knew for absolute sure that exercise would *not* affect the size or shape of your body, would you still be doing it? If you can say, 'Yes, I'd do it no matter what because it makes me feel good, it revitalises me and makes me happy,' that's fabulous! You're likely to keep doing it. But if you say through gritted teeth, 'Come what may, I *will* exercise for 30 minutes every day,' it's only a matter of time before you give up. Instead ask yourself, 'what activity can I do today that will get me moving? What body-play fits in with my plans for the day? A walk, swim, jog, weights, yoga? Dancing to a few songs while I do my housework, sprinting every time I go up stairs, playing with my kids on the lawn…?' I'm quite convinced doing 10 minutes of activity with a good feeling is (bio chemically) better for you than doing 30 minutes daily accompanied by hateful thoughts which flood you with unhealthy chemicals.

So, how do we make the mental switch from an active lifestyle being a chore to being a natural, fun part of our lives? How do we turn loathing into loving? It isn't as difficult as you think when you:
- ♥ understand your attitudes towards exercise
- ♥ encourage your MIND and body to both want exercise
- ♥ find fun ways to incorporate body-play into your life
- ♥ start loving body-play!

SELF-LOVE IS UNDERSTANDING YOUR ATTITUDE TOWARDS EXERCISE

Self♥ = recognising mental bars that keep us from being active

Ironically we often stop ourselves from being active because we've been conditioned to be ashamed of our bodies. *I was out walking when three college students walked past and the one jabbed the other and said, 'If I were that fat, I'd just stay inside.' And that's what I did; I put away my walking shoes for two years after that.* Our culture, instead of using encouraging tactics to help us participate *more*, shames us into doing *less*. Instead of an overweight person being applauded for her efforts she is subjected to cruel ridicule. Outrageous and sad. However, the more you participate in a life of action, the:

- ♥ less time you have to eat,
- ♥ the more you are out improving your metabolism so it uses up more calories,
- ♥ the more feel-good endorphins you release,
- ♥ the more energetic and vibrant you feel, and
- ♥ the less likely you are to feel down and comfort-eat!

It's societies warped messages that often land up stopping us from taking the very actions that would help us live healthier. *Many a time I have looked with longing at the water, wanting desperately to join in, but feeling too embarrassed.* If society would accept, encourage and applaud you, it would help you avoid the mental prison that has sometimes accompanied us from childhood. *I went to my dance group last night and am still euphoric today. While dancing I thought how much my time with Remix Dance Project (a combination of able-bodied dancers with disabled people) changed me. I could feel that I was accepted despite not being slim, despite not dancing well, despite often crying and being insecure. That atmosphere of acceptance and appreciation each person offered made it a spiritual experience for me. My time there made me feel I'm worth looking after and that's the antidote to self-destruction. I can expose my physical shortcomings and still be accepted. Every time I prove to myself that I'm acceptable as an adult I like myself a little more.*

Write in a journal about how your life would have been different if you could have cast aside your sense of being judged by others. What activities would you have taken part in? How would you have felt if you'd done that? How would it have helped you health wise?

Self♥ = recognising which activities you really don't like

When you dread an activity, you're doing it either to keep others off your back, or it doesn't suit you, or it has psychological hooks for you. *I don't particularly enjoy exercises like walking and treadmill and rowing. I just did them because people said they were good for me. But it was never much fun, and I couldn't wait for them to be over!* Be open to revising your attitude. It's important to be open-minded to the fact that just because you dislike some forms of activity now, that doesn't mean you always will. *Hopefully one day I'll get over my hate for walking... I suspect that as I become lighter and less constrained by my size, I will grow to enjoy other forms of exercise and sports as well.*

At the same time, holding onto knowing what *isn't* right for you in the face of opposition is just as important. *Right now, I sure as hell am not going to listen to anyone else tell me that I need to walk more to lose weight or control my diabetes. I will not walk. For now, I'll do it when I have to, like in shopping malls or around work. But I definitely won't do it as formal exercise and I'm definitely not doing it for fun.* To many this may sound like the voice of someone stubbornly refusing to do what she *should* be doing. Not so! This pilgrim is honouring her wisdom about not doing something that she knows is unsustainable because it's not enjoyable. This is someone assertively stating her needs – drum rolls and applause for her. Way too many Dietonians have been steam-rollered into doing things they don't want to in the name of keeping others happy. In the process, they've become caught up in the vicious cycle of starting something, discontinuing it, then feeling like a failure.

Make a list of all the activities you currently don't like and why you don't like them, e.g. walking, because my legs chafe; or jogging because the tendon under my foot is tight. At the end, please conclude with this sentence: 'I am receptive to enjoying these activities in the future.

Self♥ = listening, to learn which activities *are* right for *you*

Learn to choose what's right for you, both from a body and a mind point of view. *Swimming is good for me – physically and emotionally. It comes naturally. Swimming has never made me feel pain or like crying. In a pool a heavy person isn't limited or held back by size or weight. Ah, water, it is so liberating.*

When you buy into the 'no pain, no gain' baloney, you aren't listening to your body. Stretching your body is one thing, but being in pain is another. *When running a steep hill or getting tired, I used to tell myself I must suffer for all the damage I've done to myself. Thoughts like 'no pain, no gain' used to occupy my mind all the way. Now I run at a slow pace, and take leisurely walks in-between, and enjoy it! As soon as I start thinking I must do that extra push to feel the buurrrnn, I remind myself of the reasons I'm doing exercise ... health and fun!*

You may have so many conditioned ideas about exercise, you're quite sure you hate every last exercise option there is. There must be one activity you don't hate. *Exercise seems the most difficult thing in the world to do. I danced a bit by myself yesterday morning. I think that might just be the one exercise that I will be able to do and not hate.*

Self ♥ = knowing your preferences

Structured body play may be what you most enjoy. *"I prefer the structured work-out of a gym as I seem to push myself harder in an exercise class with other members."* For others, structure is an absolute turn-off: *"I don't really want to learn steps or any martial stuff, it's too structured for me, I just want to move and explore. Anything that even vaguely looks like something that belongs in a gym makes me want to run in the opposite direction."* And maybe what suits you is just silly fun: *"Formal exercise doesn't work for me. But I love to dance, so I dance with my broom, I do upward jumps with my feather duster, and I waltz with my vacuum cleaner".*

"Your body doesn't reject silly fun, it revels in it! Promise! And the bonus of dancing to housework is that you're multi-tasking in a healthy way: *"I used to plop down in front of the TV and doze through most of the programs. Now if I want to watch TV, I do something active at the same time. I lie on the carpet and do leg lifts, or a hold onto the back of the couch and do some stretching, or do push-ups against a wall. I'm stretching and toning and staying awake to see my favorite programs too."* The whole point is that there is no real right or wrong way – just a way that works best for you and your lifestyle.

Exercising our own power of choice, not someone else's (a husband's, lover's, father's, mother's, siblings, friends) is ultimately what matters. It may feel like I'm belabouring this point, but it is difficult for the average Dietonian who is desperate to do simply anything to lose weight, and who is constantly being told she makes bad choices, to hold onto what she knows is right for her in the face of others who issue forth (often uninvited) ideas on exercise programs: what kind, how much and at what speed or intensity. *"I so enjoyed my dancing this morning - it makes the day a lot more enjoyable when there is no pressure with regard to how long or how far (like there would be if I went for a walk or cycled). In fact I had to remind myself not to carry on too long or I would have been late for work."*

Make a list of all the kinds of activities you either know you love to do as well as those you remember loving to do. Which of them would give you pleasure to start doing now even if it's in a limited way? And if you can't think of any – then ask yourself what is blocking you from knowing.

SELF-LOVE IS ENCOURAGING YOUR MIND AND BODY TO WANT EXERCISE

Self♥ = visualising exercise as something positive

For exercise to become something positive, a mental shift is necessary. This cannot happen if what you're doing makes you groan and think of all sorts of excuses not to do it. *Last year I truly felt that I was never ever going to be thin, so I might as well give up on that idea and accept being fat. This year I feel differently... there's a shift in my thinking. Lately I have visions of strength and power and agility. I don't want to be a super-athlete or to compete with anyone. I just want to compete with myself. I have visions of swimming longer, harder, faster...* This body pilgrim has changed the possibilities in her life – which include slimming down – but without pressurising herself. She has started thinking of exercise not as a means to get thin but as a way to feel strong, powerful and agile. *That's* seeing exercise positively!

What visions could you hold about exercising that would spur you one? PS Being thin isn't one of them; it's a side effect of, not the reason for, being active.

Self♥ = growing your 'want' power

When we started dancing in the The Joy-Filled Body play group yesterday, I felt so physically constrained. I actually felt that I was physically disabled and that it was impossible for me to do the kind of dancing and movement that I really wanted to. But inside of me there was a voice crying out to dance, crying out to be freed to move the way she really wants to move. I felt so helpless, because I didn't know how to free her. I realized that I needed to start listening to the inner me, the one whose dreams were crushed by reality/life/my own actions and/or lack of faith. So I'm listening now. And right now the voice is saying 'Swim and dance. Swim and dance. Set me free.' As Dietonians, we are so used to the advice of others that we seldom listen to ourselves. But when you do tune into your own wisdom and act out what your body wants, you're doing what's right for it.

Self-love is building that 'want' power by reminding yourself about how good you felt during those times when your body was active. *My body has been craving exercise (I used to attend gym, then tore ligaments and besides doing my own housework the only other exercise I get is jumping to conclusions). Some mornings I wake up after having dreamt that I've exercised and I feel absolutely great (the power of the mind is amazing). I think back to 2001 when I was 88llbs lighter and fitter, and did a 30 mile walk. It really felt good to be fit and in control of my weight.*

But you're one of those Dietonians who can't think of a time in your adulthood when exercise made you feel great. . . Then cast your mind back to your childhood. *Do you know what I miss about being physically fit? The power, freedom and strength. Remember when you could run fast, and swim hard, and jump high? I long to be able to move freely.*

Right now, make a list of what you miss about being fit. What do you long to be able to do without effort in your body?

We can also boost our 'want' power by reminding ourselves what it is we *don't* want.
I'm so tired of being tired. Sometimes I feel out of breath and sometimes my bones and muscles feel very weary. I don't want to continue like this. It's also about realizing that it's more painful to stay where you are than to change. *For me, the risks of remaining as I am are too high, and too painful. Caterpillar to butterfly. Bud to flower. Oh, it so is time for change in my life...*
Rather forget about being fit for weight-loss purposes and focus instead on health gain and the multiple other benefits of living actively. *I can't say exercise is my thing, but I have to admit that I love that glowing feeling when I stop. So I concentrate on how I'll feel afterwards rather than how I'm feeling now.*

I really testify to the fact that when I exercise, the endorphins help to give me a positive outlook.

I could never be an exercise bunny, but walking on the beach puts me into a meditative trance; I can walk a long time and feel at peace.

As I walk, I play these pictures over and over in my head of my cells becoming healthier and flushing out toxins.

I'm definitely less constipated when I walk a lot.

I found that just wriggling and fidgeting while sitting watching TV energized me.

I felt so refreshed after the swim and so revitalised that I slept like a baby because I was tired and not lazy.

My joints would prefer not to have to carry that extra weight.

Exercise can be a good stress-reliever – perhaps that would in turn make me want less sugar?

My goal is to increase my fitness levels, and the best part is that my blood glucose control will be better too, because exercise increases insulin sensitivity, oh yeah!

Recognise what research is now highlighting: fitness and feeling positive about yourself are more important to your health than fatness. *Every year magazine Heart and Soul has a competition to find a woman for their cover who is full-figured and fit. Their point is that you can be fat and fit. Now, granted, not all fat women are fit. But then again, not all thin women are fit either. So my goal is to become fit. And maybe that will mean I'll become slender.*

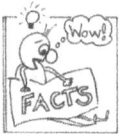

William L Haskell, professor emeritus of medicine at the Stanford Center for Research in Disease Prevention (USA) agrees. After reviewing 12 studies conducted at research clinics to determine the relative roles of fitness and fatness in the development of heart disease and diabetes, this was his opinion: 'If you have trouble losing weight, don't give up on physical activity, because being active and overweight is better than being overweight and inactive.

Read up on the benefits of exercise and make as long a list as possible of how it could benefit *your* personal health.

Self♥ = awakening old dreams

Reawakening old dreams is a great way to rekindle the excitement you once felt for something. *When I was in my late teens I promised myself that when I was thinner, I would join a modern dance or jazz dance class. But I became fatter, and the dream of dancing became a distant memory, until yesterday, when that dream was reawakened at our dance group. Oh the possibility of it all.* You don't have to bury your dreams – they'll always be there, just waiting to be unearthed. Keeping your dreams alive breeds hope and excitement. *In Michael Jackson's song 'Keep the Faith' he sings about the dreams you share with no-one else because they seem so silly, so far out. Being a dancer has been that kind of dream for me. It was/is my fantasy career. I don't want to be a professional dancer, but I do want to dance, for the sheer fun of it."*

SELF-LOVE IS INCORPORATING BODY-PLAY INTO YOUR LIFE

Self♥ = overcoming limitations

Get mentally fitter about getting your body fitter. *They say your mind can take you beyond the limits your body may place on you – the difference between dropping out of the race and finishing an ultra Marathon is a mental one.* It also takes mental preparation to change the way you tackle incorporating body-play into your life. It's often that mental preparation that determines whether you grow in love with body-play or whether you continue to hate exercise. *Who can truly put limits on myself except for me?* Mentally 'seeing' the vision you have for the new fit and healthy you is also important. *In a pool I am strong and graceful and I can move... When I swim freestyle lengths, I feel such power as my arms slice through the water – one, two, three ... ten!*

You can just visualise this escaping Dietonian! Remember that the brain cannot tell the difference between what is real and what is imagined, so bio chemically your body recreates positive neuropeptides every time you mentally run those pictures through your brain. With each rehearsal, you help build a new neural pathway, creating cells with more receptor sites to receive these positive neuropeptides. And if doing a single big block of body-play seems too tough, make it feel easier to tackle; break it into smaller chunks. *The idea of doing 30 minutes of exercise a day was off-putting; it depressed me and seemed like such a big challenge. When I broke it into smaller amounts I found it mentally so much easier to get started. I like doing 10 minutes before breakfast, 10 minutes at lunch and 10 minutes before supper – that's much more do-able for me. So I'm still doing my 30 minutes of exercise a day, just not all at once. And the bonus is, I get to feel successful three times in a day!*

Others prefer simply to build up the exercise slowly. *I started off doing just five minutes a day. Doing such small amounts was really easy. Then I extended it by just three minutes per day each week. Now I'm doing over 20 minutes a day and finding it's mentally and physically easy and I'm enjoying it.*

Self♥ = being open-minded

Even though you will sometimes recognise that an activity you like has physical limitations for you at your current size, be prepared to give it an open-minded try because it can become a motivating start-up factor. *The class I went to this morning has been a catalyst. It's as if I awakened from a catatonic state and now I want to be free to move more.* For you the catalyst could be Pilates or yoga or hiking. We're all unique.

What might you like to experiment with? Find out what activities are in your neighbourhood and see if you can attend a once-off session to evaluate if it's for you. This way you have no need to sign up for something you might hate. Be open-minded about it and ask yourself, what am I enjoying about this and what am I not? Does this make me feel joyful and revitalised? Would I want to do it again without someone nagging me?

You could even experiment with combining two activities and find that certain combinations work for you. *I feel vulnerable about dancing, because my movement out of water is limited. Maybe, for now, I should dance in the water.*

Do you enjoy walking but would love to be able to jog? How about walking 100 paces and then running 50, and gradually changing the ratio as you get fitter? If you love to go on walks out in nature, what about hiking? Do you love to window-shop or look at beautiful gardens? Then why not walk or roller-blade past shop windows or in a beautiful residential area?

SELF-LOVE IS DOING WHAT IS SUSTAINABLE

Self♥ = doing wannas

When you have 'want' power, you stay active, not because you 'hafta' but because you 'wanna.' There's a vast different between wannas and haftas.

121

Wannas use up less mental energy doing, and their exercise is thus vastly more sustainable than haftas. It's of no use whatsoever taking up an exercise regime if you hate it; unless you have an iron will, it's unsustainable from the start. *I hate walking and joining a walking club made it even worse. Although I could clearly see the effects physically – improved blood glucose control, increased fitness, looser clothes – the emotional price was high. I hated going so much... sometimes I cried when I got home. I just felt so hopeless. After a few weeks the walking became easier but I still didn't enjoy it, and eventually I left.*

Contrast this lack of energy and motivation with the vibrancy of this next wanna. *Dancing! Yip, I love that. I'd go to raves and dance for ten hours non-stop! I love the way the music breaks down and builds up and the amazing beat! It's awesome! The atmosphere is like a huge surge of adrenaline. You can feel the beat under your feet and the base hits your body with an incredible energy!* Sustainability is determined, though, not just by how much you want to do something but also by other factors.

Self♥ = avoiding injury

With every new diet – a new running program. I usually ended up injuring a muscle because of overdoing it.
*

Self♥ = using the right equipment or clothing

It was a pain having to change into special tennis clothes. I've taken up brisk walking instead, and simply pop my walking shoes in my car so I can pull them on at anytime.

(Having said that, *don't* invest in expensive equipment until you're absolutely sure that what you're thinking of taking up is a 'wanna.')

Self♥ = making allowance for the seasonality of activities

The weather impacting on your body-play will need to include an alternative activity upfront that you know you can fall back on. *I know I won't swim at home in winter because it's too cold – I'm going to have to find an indoor pool or find another activity.*

Make a list of all the factors that would make body-play sustainable for you. What factors take away from that?

Self♥ = setting realistic goals and affirming them

While you're busy keeping your dreams alive, do be sure also to keep yourself firmly grounded in your current reality. *The kind of dancing where dancers fly (literally) across a room may not be possible right now given my size and weight, but I'm going to get there. I'm thinking before I'm 35 I want to be able to do the kind of dancing that took place in the last scene of Dirty Dancing. That gives me five years.*

Don't allow your size to stop you from dreaming but do set yourself a realistic time-frame in which to accomplish your dream. Then set yourself smaller goals that lead up to your bigger goal. *My aim is to have the confidence to take dance lessons and to dance even twice a week.* Then, keep affirming that your belief is possible to maintain. *I believe it's possible – I'm going to be a dancing queen! ♫♪♫ You can dance, you can dance, Having the time of your lives ... See that girl, watch that scene, Digging the dancing queen ♫♪♫ (Abba)*

What is stopping you? How can you take one step today, even a really small one, towards your dreams?

Self♥ = is choosing healthy role-models

Find yourself positive role-models. The actions of those you admire can inspire and motivate you. Role-models remind you of what you long to do and fill you with hope. You can also be a role-model to others if you act out of enjoyment and a lack of self-consciousness. *Today at the dance group, there were two women who were especially graceful. What I admired most was their lack of self-consciousness. I was filled with a longing to be able to dance like that. Both of them were older, grey-haired women and yet, their range of movement was fantastic. It got me thinking – if women in their 50s could dance like that, what's to stop me?*

Self♥ = being self-forgiving

Usual Dietonian thinking is that you need to stick rigidly to your exercise regime and if you don't, you should feel guilty and punish yourself by doing double to make up for it. But the average Dietonian is already so saddled with this black-and-white thinking and the resultant guilt that the feelings of helplessness and despair grow instead with you giving up on getting fitter. It's far healthier to recognise that sometimes life gets in the way of your plans. Instead of beating yourself up for not achieving what you'd set out to do,

123

simply acknowledge that things didn't go exactly as planned, and continue making your progress, guilt-free. *I really want to cycle every day but I also know that is not always realistic. Sometimes things crop up or the weather is foul, and feeling guilty about not cycling just because I promised myself I would is not helping.*

It's not only that life steps in; we sometimes land up doing things we wish we hadn't, then adopting black-and-white ways of thinking. *I'm quite sensitive to rich and creamy food. But, too late, she cried! I don't even feel like any sort of exercise because healthy food and exercise go hand in hand, not chocolate and exercise.* Note that if you continue on your path despite the missteps, you're making progress. Focusing on what you *are* achieving and on where you're intending to get to rather than dashing your hopes every time you slip is far more helpful and healthful. *The old me would have said, 'Well, I ruined all the benefits of swimming this morning with my binge tonight.' But that was in the days when I was exercising to lose weight. Now it's because I love swimming. And so I'll keep swimming even when I binge.*

What are you already doing that you can focus on more strongly? Where do you need to stop belittling your efforts?

SELF-LOVE IS LOVING BODY-PLAY

Self♥ = increasing your body-fun in non-painful ways.

To achieve your dreams of enjoying being active, you may first have to work on slowly increasing activity within your own limits. *It feels so amazing when I'm in the water and I'm pushing myself harder... This afternoon in the pool I felt a burst of energy, and decided to try for three consecutive lengths instead of two, and then once I completed three, I told myself to try for four, and that if I couldn't make it, I could always stop halfway in the pool. But I made it! In the words of L'Oreal: I swim ... because I'm worth it.*

The swim at gym this morning was so great that I'm thinking of swimming again tonight. I'm not telling myself I must swim, I'll see how I feel tonight. Swimming twice in one day that will be a first for me. The last time I did that was when I was a teenager.

I'm really unfit, so it's no use starting something that is going to make me so stiff I can't move – that's enough to make me give up fast. So I've had to develop patience and realize my body can't go from zero to hero in one fell swoop. I started with five minutes of walking, which I increased to seven and later to ten minutes. Then I started doing it more often. This has worked so much better than previous times when I've started overzealously, only to give it up because I hated it.

Self ♥ = knowing your preferences

Structured body play may be what you most enjoy. *"I prefer the structured work-out of a gym as I seem to push myself harder in an exercise class with other members."* For others, structure is an absolute turn-off: *"I don't really want to learn steps or any martial stuff, it's too structured for me, I just want to move and explore. Anything that even vaguely looks like something that belongs in a gym makes me want to run in the opposite direction."* And maybe what suits you is just silly fun: *"Formal exercise doesn't work for me. But I love to dance, so I dance with my broom, I do upward jumps with my feather duster, and I waltz with my vacuum cleaner".* "Your body doesn't reject silly fun, it revels in it! Promise! And the bonus of dancing to housework is that you're multi-tasking in a healthy way: *"I used to plop down in front of the TV and doze through most of the programs. Now if I want to watch TV, I do something active at the same time. I lie on the carpet and do leg lifts, or a hold onto the back of the couch and do some stretching, or do push-ups against a wall. I'm stretching and toning and staying awake to see my favorite programs too."* The whole point is that there is no real right or wrong way – just a way that works best for you and your lifestyle.

Exercising our own power of choice, not someone else's (a husband's, lover's, father's, mother's, siblings, friends) is ultimately what matters. It may feel like I'm belabouring this point, but it is difficult for the average Dietonian who is desperate to do simply anything to lose weight, and who is constantly being told she makes bad choices, to hold onto what she knows is right for her in the face of others who issue forth (often uninvited) ideas on exercise programs: what kind, how much and at what speed or intensity. *"I so enjoyed my dancing this morning - it makes the day a lot more enjoyable when there is no pressure with regard to how long or how far (like there would be if I went for a walk or cycled). In fact I had to remind myself not to carry on too long or I would have been late for work."*

Make a list of all the kinds of activities you either know you love to do as well as those you remember loving to do once upon a time when you were younger or fitter. Which of them would give you pleasure to start doing now even if it's in a limited way? And if you can't think of any – then ask yourself what is blocking you from knowing.

Self ♥ = knowing your preferences

Structured body play may be what you most enjoy. *"I prefer the structured work-out of a gym as I seem to push myself harder in an exercise class with other members."* For others, structure is an absolute turn-off: *"I don't really want to learn steps or any martial stuff, it's too structured for me, I just want to move and explore. Anything that even vaguely looks like something that belongs in a gym makes me want to run in the opposite direction."* And maybe what suits you is just silly fun: *"Formal exercise doesn't work for me. But I love to dance, so I dance with my broom, I do upward jumps with my feather duster, and I waltz with my vacuum cleaner".* "Your body doesn't reject silly fun, it revels in it! Promise! And the bonus of dancing to housework is that you're multi-tasking in a healthy way: *"I used to plop down in front of the TV and doze through most of the programs. Now if I want to watch TV, I do something active at the same time. I lie on the carpet and do leg lifts, or a hold onto the back of the couch and do some stretching, or do push-ups against a wall. I'm stretching and toning and staying awake to see my favorite programs too."* The whole point is that there is no real right or wrong way – just a way that works best for you and your lifestyle.

Self♥= increasing your body-fun in non-painful ways.

To reach your dreams of living enjoying being active, you may have to first work on slowly increasing your activity within your own limits so as not to injure yourself. *"It feels so amazing when I'm in the water and I'm pushing myself harder.. This afternoon I felt a burst of energy, and decided to try for 3 consecutive lengths instead of 2, and then once I completed 3, I told myself to try for 4, and that if I couldn't make it, I could always stop halfway in the pool. But I made it, I made it! Yeah! "In my younger days I could swim lengths for an hour without stopping/resting for a break. Imagine that! In the words of L'Oreal - I swim ... "Because I'm worth it."* As this morsel indicates you need to:
- ♥ listen to your body do more when it feels right
- ♥ work in harmony with your body by preparing yourself mentally;
- ♥ not set you up for failure;
- ♥ pat you on the back for even the smallest victories.
- ♥ keep a vision of what was once possible for you:
- ♥ find quotes and sayings that motivate and inspire you:

126

Increase the duration, intensity or frequency of your body-play as it feels intuitively right for you to: *The swim at gym this morning was so great that I'm thinking of swimming tonight again. I'm not telling myself I MUST swim. I want to but I'll see how I feel tonight. That will be a first for me - swimming twice in one day. The last time I did that was when I was a teenager.* Whatever you do, don't do too much too soon – your mind and body need time to make both adjustments. Rather start off really slowly and then build it up: *I'm really unfit, so it's no use starting something that is going to make me so stiff I can't move – that's enough to make me give up fast. So I've had to develop patience and realize my body can't go from zero to hero in one foul swoop. It's better for me to start off slowly, enjoy it and be able to sustain it. So, I started with 5 minutes of walking which I then increased to 7 and later 10 minutes and then I started doing it more often too. This has worked so much better than previous times when I've started over-zealously only to give it up because I hated it.*

Self♥ = making your dreams more concrete

Writing down your goal and sharing it with supportive others makes your dream more concrete. *They say goals are dreams written down, dreams put into action. So I'm sharing the goal of my swimming with you guys, in writing.* This pilgrim not only writes down her goal but also has two forthcoming events to inspire and keep her motivated. *My goal with the swimming is twofold: to increase my fitness levels so that by the time I go overseas in June, I will be able to walk around with greater ease; to improve my HbA1C (it's a test for the three-month average of your blood sugars) in February.* Then she does something designed to reaffirm for her the immediate benefits of her swimming. *Tomorrow I'm going to test myself immediately after swimming. I just need to see for myself once again the effect that swimming has on my blood glucose control. I think it will motivate me to see a reading under 7 afterwards.* She is thinking long term, all the while remembering it's the actions she takes in the short term that count from one day to the next.

Remind yourself of the personal benefits you'll gain from doing more body-play plus all the reasons you want to continue doing it regularly. *I've been thinking about how being active has made me feel excited and positive about my future. I actually want to be around to experience all that my life is meant to be. I don't want to miss out on all God has planned for me. It's an amazing feeling to WANT to take care of myself.*

What *one* body-play activity will you commit to doing tomorrow? List all the things you'd be able to do if you were fitter.

Self♥ = lowering your standards

In the Mind over Fatter online group, during all of our discussions about body-play, there were a few of us (myself included) who admitted to not dancing because we didn't believe we danced well enough. But wise thinking can help shift your thinking: *I believe everyone can dance, it's our birthright You might think you 'can't dance' but maybe you're coming up with a whole new style and brand of dancing. Have music? Have motion? That's dance!* Who says that if I dance like an erratic windmill I'm not busy coming up with the next big rave that may sweep the world? Think about it, every single new dance form came out of someone not doing what was the prevailing thing to do. And even if I'm not – so what if I don't move like anyone else does? As young children we weren't self-conscious; we brimmed with confidence. We need to drop the conditioned standards (our psychological hooks) that stop us from indulging in body fun. *I used to think that how well I did exercise made a difference. But I've discovered my body doesn't know the difference between a waltz executed perfectly and a waltz just done for the fun of it. Once I took away the pressure to do it properly, I found it more pleasurable.* It's not a competition to do it better; it's a road to feeling healthy, alive and invigorated. Sitting on the sidelines wishing you could participate won't get you anywhere. *In the words of Lee Ann Womack's song, 'I Hope you Dance':* ♫♪♫ *And when you get the choice to sit it out or dance, I hope you dance, I hope you dance.*♫♪♫

Self♥ = raising your standards

Raise your standards in that you will only do what's fun and enjoyable. If it's silly fun, all the better! *One thing I do for body-fun is teach spinning at 5am (insane, I know!). I do it for the ability to lose myself in the music. I put the music on as loud as I can and mimic the words, like I'm on stage and doing this amazing show for a huge crowd of adoring fans! I know it's silly, but it's so much fun!*

Yes, make it psychologically legal to turn exercise into something that has all the elements of fun, play and laughter. *I just had to share with you the mad fun I had in the pool yesterday. We laughed so hard we were practically in tears. We played volleyball and we had races. The people who lost had to do star jumps in the pool or run around the pool circumference in the water. We were acting like children but who cares? It was too much fun.*

Isn't there something downright crazy about living in a culture that makes us feel apologetic about having too much fun?

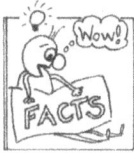

If you want to gain an additional edge in your weight war, try exercising your sense of humour. Scientists have found that 10–15 minutes of genuine giggling can burn off the amount of calories found in a medium square of chocolate! That's not all. Participants shown video clips of the 'Cosby Show' by researchers at Vanderbilt University (Nashville, Tennessee), burned up 20% more calories laughing than when they watched landscapes with sheep. Researchers calculated that laughing for 10–15 minutes a day burns up to 50 calories daily and could result in people losing 4lbs a year! [32]

In terms of your body's chemistry, laughing releases endorphins that are great for your health. Laughter is fabulous medicine. But don't laugh to lose weight – laugh because it feels great, because it's healthy for you and simply because we take ourselves *way* too seriously. It's time we lightened up.

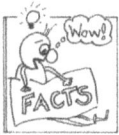

Research conducted at Graz University in Austria showed that when one group did only movement exercises while the other did 'laughter' yoga, those engaging in laughter lowered their blood pressure and recovered from strokes. The mood improved in both groups, but more noticeably so in the laughter group. Participants also said they felt 'more awake' and 'less stressed. [33]

Go on, I dare you! See if you can get to be accused of being childish (interpret that in your mind as 'childlike'). Get overly excited about little things; listen to your instinctual urges. Jump into piles of leaves, dash around mud puddles, and skip along pavements, get down on your belly to crawl alongside ants, run to find the end of the rainbow. . . It's when you access this sense of childlike play that you release frustrations and negative feelings and live a more spontaneous life.

You may play golf, tennis, hockey, netball … but unless it's a fun impromptu game in which the score doesn't count, those aren't play activities, they're competitive games. They have strict rules, with sides, and winners and losers. There is often tension, skill expectation, disappointment and criticism. It's not that they're bad; they simply aren't play. If you make time to fit play into your life, it costs nothing but it can change your life. Play is about an *attitude*. If running a marathon or gymming really hard can bring you fun and enjoyment, then it can be play for you.

Chapter 7

♥

The what, when and how to of eating

When you think about it, eating is a rather remarkable activity. We take an object that exists outside of us; put it in our mouths and chew on it, and swallow it so that some part of it literally becomes us. (Anon)

Finally ... food. Now, I'm willing to bet many of you are wondering why this chapter comes last. Usually it would come first, or the entire book would be devoted to the subject of food. Simply put, if your problem was a simple matter of dealing with the 'food' and 'eating' parts of Diet City, I wouldn't need to write this book.

So…'You are what you eat,' right? Well, yes, partly. But you are also '*how* you eat.' The The Joy-Filled Body journey is about developing a self-loving MINDset and going back to what you once did naturally. That is your starting point rather than the food itself. Having a self-loving attitude helps you implement the practical 'how to' approaches towards food and eating, enabling you to adopt new attitudes and actions with spontaneous willingness (what I refer to as 'want' power) rather than willpower.

I remember being on radio on International Non-Diet Day, when a listener phoned in sputtering with indignation, reacting the way many people do when they hear about the idea of giving up dieting. 'Pig out, tuck in?! And you're trying to tell me *that's* the way to lose weight?' However, when I say 'stop dieting' I'm not saying 'pig out'. Our experiences of trying to follow unnatural diets only to fail – then 'pig out' – mean we've forgotten there is a more balanced place between stuffing and starving.

Let's face it, how do we keep on doing the same thing over and over but expect a different result? Have you tried the Cabbage Soup diet? The Grapes only detox? The Low-carb High-protein diet that tells you to cut out fruit completely and eat more meat? The Meals in a Milkshake diet? The Apples for Two Days, Chicken for Two Days diet? Have you tried to eat like people from biblical times or excluded foods according to your blood type or body shape, or followed the supposed eating plan of a film star from a magazine? Next, have you tried more than one of the above?

Most of us have become so desperate to feel happy with our bodies; we can't help hoping the next crazy eating plan will work better than the last one. You can never reach Nature's Valley by following an eating plan or dieting because they only give you another set of rules, external to you, and disrespecting and ignoring your body needs. *The best way to feel comfortable in your body is to change what you do and start loving yourself.*

Being diet crazy is not only about food restriction. It's about your tendency to pressurise yourself to lose weight within an artificial time span. The Joy-Filled Body is very different – it's more like a long walk to freedom. As one body pilgrim realized: *The most difficult thing for me was to shed my ideas about weighing a certain amount by a certain date. When I looked back at my history, it was amazing to notice that I was constantly dieting for some event. It's taken me 30 years to get the body I have and realistically it's not going to take me three months to get it back to where I want it to be.*

The Joy-Filled Body isn't about losing 40lbs by your daughter's wedding or your next high school reunion. Instead, it's about honouring your body needs and allowing your body to arrive eventually at a place that feels natural and right for it. And that may take time.

Adding to the craziness are a whole lot of figures drawn up from selected research and averages – like BMI's and goal weights – which cannot take into account each individual's body, situation and lifestyle. Charts and tables cannot tell you what your natural weight is; only your body can. And it can only do this when you follow a self-loving enough path to have a healthy, normal and consistent eating pattern – while having a fun and active lifestyle – over a sustained period of time. Your natural body weight won't necessarily match your supposed 'goal weight' but it will be a weight and shape that is uniquely your own.

Self ♥ = listening and legalizing

To reach your natural size, you have to become body-wise. You need to listen to your body. The Joy-Filled Body path varies vastly from your average diet because the only 'rules' you'll be asked to follow are those made by your body. Instead of having an eating plan that dictates you have to eat 'x amount of x at x time', I want you to discover for yourself what works best for your body and respond accordingly. Some people are breakfast people, others aren't. Some want to be vegetarians, others don't. Each of you has your own preferences and needs, and the closer your own plan blends in with those, the more chance you have of reaching Nature's Valley because you'll be doing what you 'wanna-do' (fuelling your 'want' power) instead of what you feel you 'hafta-do' (reliant on willpower).

With all the conditioning we've been exposed to, many of us may have forgotten our bodies even have a voice. But they do! And when you relearn how to 'hear' it, it will always 'speak' to you. Once you re-access your body's wisdom, you put it in charge of helping you eat in relaxed and natural ways without insane eating plans or damaging diet products. When your choices are body-driven, you respond to your internal biological health needs rather than society's external aesthetic needs.

To reach your natural size, you must *legalize*! Food must take its rightful place…just a part of living. Food is fuel; it is essential for nutrients, for health and to stay alive. But when you react to the psychological hooks, it can feel as if food is your enemy. It's the feelings of deprivation and restriction you have to guard against. Once you take care of those, you stop obsessing about food. Self-loving actions are to legalize food, eat with enjoyment and listen to what your body is telling you. Then food starts falling into its rightful place – as a fuel for life. Your conversations change too. One Mind over Fatter group member put it this way: *I was just thinking that if a newcomer to our online support group reads many of our mails they might wonder, But where's the food/fat/weight talk? Because we talk about so many other things. Food is no longer the huge issue it was to me. I am still not eating 100% healthily, but I don't agonise about it or spend time longing for food. Now, if I want something, I simply have it and then it's over. No big deal.*

There are basically eight interconnected self ♥ing paths to improving your relationship with food:

- ♥ eating only for tummy hunger
- ♥ legalizing all eating activities (including all food)
- ♥ choosing body foods
- ♥ overcoming overeating
- ♥ beating sneak-eating
- ♥ staying calm around food
- ♥ practising self-loving ways
- ♥ coping with 'slips, dips and dives'.

The following morsels, shared by body pilgrims about how to eat the Mind over Fatter body-wise way, are designed to trigger ideas about what might work for you so that you never have to diet again. You see you're unique – so this is not a one-plan-fits-all approach. We give you guidelines and then you see how you can adapt them to fit into your life instead of trying to get your life to fit around something that's artificial.

SELF-LOVE IS EATING ONLY FOR TUMMY HUNGER

Self ♥ = becoming intimate with your various hungers

It only takes a few seconds to ascertain your body's needs and whether you are hungry or being fooled by imposter hungers. As I explained in the Mind over Fatter program, we have four kinds of hungers:

- ♥ A throat hunger: your body is signaling it's thirsty and needs liquid (preferably water).
- ♥ A head hunger: your body is signaling your mind needs distracting.
- ♥ A heart hunger: your body is signaling you want to eat for emotional reasons (you're feeling mad, bad, sad or glad or any other emotion).
- ♥ A tummy hunger: your body is hungry and is asking for food. The only real hunger of the four is tummy hunger; the rest are imposter hungers.

Sit quietly, run your tongue around your mouth and ask, 'Mouth, are you hungry or possibly thirsty?' Then place your hand on your throat and ask it, 'Are you hungry or thirsty?' If you get a 'yes' to either of these questions, your body is thirsty – it's asking for liquid, not food. This is a throat hunger. If you get a 'no' then place your hand above your navel and ask, 'Tummy, are you hungry?' If the answer is 'no', your body is not asking for food – it's an impostor hunger from either your heart or head. An impostor hunger is when either your heart or your head is 'hungry' but your body isn't. Remember that the only 'right' time to eat is when your stomach is physically hungry.

Most Dietonians have lost touch with eating for tummy hunger. *It made sense that we have different kinds of hunger and that most of them are impostor hungers that don't need food at all. Before I was given the tools to 'hear' and respond to my body's needs, I ate for a myriad reasons but seldom for physical (tummy) hunger. I found out that every other time, my body stored this food as fat because it didn't need it.*

Once I became tuned into my different kinds of hunger, it became easier for me to be conscious of when I was eating for the wrong reasons. Only then could I consciously exercise my power of choice not to feed non-physical hungers with food ... to make better choices for myself.

Self ♥ = understanding your cravings

Cravings are when you have a strong desire for a specific food rather than eating in general, and they can be either biological or psychological. Sometimes, in response to hormonal changes or a dropping blood sugar, your brain sends you signals in the form of cravings for specific food types, so in the biological sense your body is hungry for something it feels it's lacking, although your stomach isn't asking for food in general. *I'm starting to realize how much influence my body sugar levels have on my moods and behaviour. I'm pre-diabetic and when my sugar drops, I become extremely irritable. Often in eating my little bit of 'comfort-food', I'm balancing my sugar levels in my blood, and allowing myself to think clearly – it's a bit like self-care for me!*

But some 'cravings' have a psychological base: *When my father died, I couldn't stop eating peanut butter and syrup sandwiches. I used to spend hours with my father in his workshop and every break; I'd make us peanut butter and syrup sandwiches which we dunked into our coffee. It was my way of trying to reconnect with him.*

How do you know if it's a craving?
♥ Is your strong desire to eat a *particular* food?
♥ Does it seem to pop out of nowhere?
♥ Does it seem very insistent

Responding to cravings in a conscious way prevents them from escalating into a binge: *When I'm craving for something sweet, fruit just does not help! I have a packet of jelly babies in my drawer and when the sweet cravings hit, I take one. I savor it; I suck all the sugar off, and then let the jelly melt in my mouth. It takes me about five minutes to eat one. And then I reassess my cravings – am I still craving sugar? Most of the time I only need to have one or two pieces before the craving has gone.*

And sometimes, simply changing your environment gives your cravings the space to abate on their own: *We went away on holiday with friends who are total health nuts. Can you believe it; they didn't even take a packet of cookies? I was way too embarrassed to haul out my stash, so it stayed hidden. After eating properly for only a few days, I found I had so much more energy and I didn't have to take laxatives. After two weeks with these friends, my sugar cravings had disappeared and it almost seemed normal to nibble on a carrot. Talk about going cold turkey!*

Cravings can become habitual. Biologically, the more sugar you eat, the more your body creates receptors for the sugar, and the more you heighten your sugar 'threshold'. This simply means that you need more sugar to perceive the same sweetness.

Cravings are psychological when they are linked to a particular event or person, or when they point to something going on in your life.

- ♥ Craving oily food? What needs to be oiled/greased in your life?
- ♥ Craving solid food? Where in your life are you not feeling substantial enough?
- ♥ Craving sweetness? Where does your life need sweetening?

If you find yourself craving one particular kind of food, ask yourself: Why this food?

- ♥ Is there a memory connected to this food?
- ♥ Is this a food that is 'illegal' and I want it because I can't have it?

Self♥ = knowing your impostor hungers

We eat for habitual reasons that are not connected to a physical tummy hunger; we eat to fill our physical or emotional cravings. *The other day I wanted something nice. So I asked myself are you really hungry? And I couldn't say yes, but also couldn't pinpoint this feeling I had ... Then, when I did the hunger exercise later, the word 'emptiness' struck me. I am obviously trying to fill a 'gap' with food, thinking the emptiness is hunger.*

Eating out of habit often happens under certain circumstances or in the presence of certain people. *When I get mad at my boss, I want to eat a muffin, not because suddenly I am hungry, but because I am looking to do something that will make me feel better. If I can break that habit, I will eat when I am hungry – and because everything is legal, muffins, chocs and nougat won't have more 'pull' than a carrot. Then my body will choose what it needs in that moment.*

Taking the time to ask yourself which hunger you're feeding (head, throat, heart or tummy) is enormously valuable, especially if you're prone to comfort-eating because eating for heart hungers isn't a self-loving choice in the long run. *I have found that I am no longer keeping quiet in order to keep the peace. If the decisions or actions being made are detrimental to me and my values, I will not accept them quietly anymore. The positive spin-off from this is that my binge eating has decreased, so there is definitely a connection between the emotions and comfort eating for me.*

Whenever you find yourself eating in response to an impostor hunger but you eat anyway, it's a signal to stop and delve into the attic of your emotions to see what's going on. In the following morsel, anxiety is a heart hunger: *I recently moved in to a new house. My 18-year-old brother was keeping me company, but as soon as he went back home, I become very hungry round about 9:30 at night. Asking myself the question, who is really hungry?' I found it was my heart! I was afraid of being alone in this big house. I had someone add an extra lock to my bedroom door. Now the hunger is gone!*

Body pilgrims have come up with many ways to feed impostor hungers: *I now have water when I experience those hungers, then play with my dogs, phone a friend, do my nails, or wash my hair – anything to pamper myself! And it works.*

Replacements for food? I'm thinking of becoming a mad writer! As in . . . every time I want to binge eat, I will binge write instead – replace my comfort eating with comfort writing. Wouldn't that be wild?

My ex contacted me to let me know that the dog we had together had been knocked over by a car! I cried a lot. Eventually I shared it with my new husband. He was incredible; he listened, let me cry on his shoulder and hugged me and let me just let it all out. I feel so much better about it and now can say that I have not eaten to try to stuff down the emotions!

I'm examining my relationship with my mother. I was very different to her and up until now I have tried to be like her. But now I'm allowing myself to be who I want to be, without hiding it. I want to discover what it is that truly satisfies me. I'm very surprised every time I find out that it isn't sugar!

Self♥ = responding to your real hungers

Once you know that a hunger really is a tummy (physical) hunger, the next step is to know just how hungry you are. This helps you to know when best to eat. Do this by using the Mind over Fatter rating scale.

Tummy hunger rating scale

1. I'm ravenous, even sawdust would look edible
3. I'd like to eat now (*optimal time to eat)*
5. I feel satisfied (*optimal time to stop eating)*
10. I am bursting-balloon-full

1-4 =   physical hunger reasons for eating
5-10= imposter hungers - excuses for eating

Understanding your hungers also means eating *whenever* you are hungry…but]
♥ *if you're not sure that you're physically hungry, you aren't.*
♥ if you have a tummy hunger, drinking water won't take the hunger away for long.
Think of body hunger as desirable (your friend) and not as something to avoid (your enemy).

Dietonians escaping Diet City are still programmed with old diet thinking that can block our progress and it takes time to learn to recognise your body's real signals: *I didn't know how to hear my body's hunger signals, and as a result I used to wait until I was starving before I would eat. I thought 'hungry' meant 'starving'. But now that I know how to rate my hunger, I've started eating and stopping a lot sooner.*
   We've become so conditioned to the cultural routine of breakfast, lunch and supper that the idea of eating whenever your body is hungry takes some adjusting. *When I was on diet, I was always hungry. I thought that by going hungry I was speeding up weight loss. Imagine my horror when I discovered that all I'd been doing was slowing my metabolism and making it more difficult for my body to lose weight. Now I eat whenever my BODY is asking for food. With that, my whole eating pattern has changed. I used to eat three big meals, now I eat small snacks throughout the day as I get physically hungry.* And it definitely takes a mindset of not having to wait for a set time to eat, but to eat whenever we are physically hungry. *I remember fearing not being able to eat everything I wanted to – after all, when I was listening to my body, it felt like it needed much less than what my mind thought it wanted! What helped me was reminding myself that I could eat whenever I was hungry, so if I was physically hungry 40 minutes after eating, I was allowed to eat again. That released me from waiting for mealtimes.*
   Make sure you have a plentiful stock of all the foods you like at home, at work and in a food bag (nuts, fresh or dried fruit, and jerky work well). That way, you won't ever have feelings of deprivation. Okay, so what if you are hungry but the meal isn't ready? *I find it helpful to eat something small, like a starter, when I am very hungry and the food is not 'ready' yet. For instance: a fruit, fresh veggies, or even a cup of red bush tea.*
   And what might you do if you're a nibbler? *I used to nibble continuously while cooking, and then still ate the meal because I believed that families ought to eat together. Now, if I nibble while I'm preparing a meal, I'll often just sit with them and have a cup of tea. After all, it's about being together, not necessarily about eating together that is important.*

Self♥ = expanding your awareness of your body's communication

Becoming aware of when your body is truly hungry and when not is just the beginning. By truly listening you are able to give it exactly what it needs to energize it. Your body is always talking to you, but its whisperings often aren't loud or insistent enough to penetrate your busy-ness, or you don't recognise what it is saying. *At first it was like I couldn't 'hear' anything. Then I started keeping a diary, monitoring things like when I was lethargic versus energized, and I noticed that if I was eating a lot of candy, I struggled to keep my eyes open. That was the start of 'hearing' my body. If I hadn't started some sort of monitoring system, I'd still be at Square One.*

     When your body gets really desperate, it screams – like when you're stuffed or you have such severe indigestion you can't help but notice – and that's when you usually become aware of it!

To listen to your body ask yourself:
♥ How did your body feel after you ate?
♥ Is it registering a protest about either the quantity or what you ate?
♥ If it is protesting, where are you feeling it in your body?
♥ How would your body have felt it you'd eaten less of the same food?
♥ How would it have felt if you'd eaten a different food?
♥ How would it have felt if you'd eaten a different combination?
♥ Might your body prefer to eat this food at a different time of day?

Unfortunately the body doesn't speak verbally, rather via symptoms, and you have to interpret what they mean. The symptom may be: feeling dizzy, being bloated, and feeling like you have a ball stuck in your throat, heaviness on your chest, having limbs that feel restless or lethargic, having indigestion, or a headache, or prickles. Sometimes, your body sings! *For me, salads have always been 'diet food.' But I've realized that as long as the salad isn't just lettuce, cucumber and tomato, I really enjoy them. Salads with toasted nuts, shavings of cheese, slithers of chicken or lots of herbs are yummy – they make my body sing.*

     With awareness and taking the time to tune into your body, you can actually learn what it likes or dislikes. Your body's symptoms are its feedback. *I've realized that if I eat eggs or any tomato-based dishes in the morning, I taste them all day. But if eat them for supper, I don't have the same experience. I figure it's just my body telling me what I can eat when.*

When I drink milk, I have the most dreadful postnasal drip; it's like my body is crying. But if I eat yoghurt or drink buttermilk, my body doesn't react in the same way.

If I eat white bread, my body feels bloated and if I eat candy I feel sleepy. If I overeat, my tummy feels uncomfortable."

When you tune into those symptoms, you learn to make better choices on your journey out of Diet City. *By listening to my body with different ears, I've been able to respond in ways that prevent me getting body symptoms I don't want, like indigestion or bloating. Since I've become aware of how various foods react in my body, I find myself choosing not to eat (for example) white bread, because it gives me indigestion. Because I no longer want to feel like that, it's a vastly different motivation from not being allowed to eat white bread.*

SELF-LOVE IS LEGALIZING FOOD

As with many things related to being a Dietonian, it's the ostensible 'cure' that actually causes the problem. Although our 'drug of choice' (food) is a legal one, what often causes problematic eating is that we have made many foods psychologically illegal. In Diet City there are laws against certain kinds of food and eating – it's illegal to: eat particular foods, not calorie-count, binge, or eat with enjoyment in public. These laws teach our internal voices to become critical and accept comments from 'helpful' others that let us know our behaviour is unacceptable.

But let's face it, there's something about the human spirit that reacts negatively to feeling deprived and restricted. As Dr Hawkins points out in his book *Power vs. Force*, 'allowing' and 'wanting to' result in muscles testing strong whereas 'controlling' and 'having to' make them test weak. Tell me something is forbidden and immediately it's more desirable. *I found legalizing food incredible. I couldn't bear to be told what I could and couldn't eat and when foods were forbidden. It was as if I was determined to have them. When I moved illegal foods to my 'can eat' list, I no longer craved them.*

By legalizing food, it stops pulling your attention and demanding to be eaten. *In Overcoming Overeating, they talk about 'stocking up' on foods that 'shimmer' to you – going out and purposefully buying tons of the stuff so that you can convince your body (and yourself) you're not depriving it. After a while, you find the things you bought sitting on the shelf in the cupboard, and they have totally lost their shimmer!"*

However, there is an enormous difference between something being *psychologically* legal versus being *biologically* legal. With psychologically legal foods, the psychological hooks have been removed, leading to you making better decisions because you feel as if you have choice. *People think, Wow! I can eat chocolate cake everyday! Last year when I lived alone, I would buy myself an entire chocolate cake, but having it there, all to myself, killed the desire for it. I would end up giving most of it away.*
The psychological hooks are still dictating to you if you haven't learned to make healthy choices or you're still constantly fighting thoughts of food.

Biologically, your health will suffer on loads of chocolate cake. Even though we know this, it doesn't automatically mean we'll eat less of it. But when your *attitude* towards chocolate cake changes – that you can eat it in any quantity, whenever you want to *if you wish* – that's where you make psychologically healthier choices. Legalizing food is simply a means to removing the *feeling* of being mentally restricted. It's freeing you from the guilt and shame of eating chocolate cake, and *choosing* to savor one piece.

Yes, I know! It sounds like it's all the wrong way round. But constantly banning foods and depriving yourself of them is long-term insanity, because the rebound action is to overeat and sneak-eating. The process of legalizing is like going temporarily 'insane' in order to gain long-term sanity.

The whole idea of legalizing is without doubt one of the trickiest stages for Dietonians because you are made to realize just how much conditioning you have to overcome. And, worse still, you have to adopt it in the face of cultural beliefs that overwhelmingly believe if you 'allow' overweight people to legalize food they won't be able to control themselves.

As if that obstacle isn't enough, the whole basis for legalizing rests on the belief that you can trust your body – which is a foreign concept for the average Dietonian. *As a young child I was force-fed for many years by my grandmother. I was very small-boned and she was anxious that I would starve myself to death. She taught me that my body cannot be trusted to know when I am hungry.* But just you watch people who have never had an issue with food and eating. They certainly overeat from time to time, but they don't sneak-eat and they can eat chocolate or ice-cream without feeling guilt. *My friend is slender, but she comfort-eats occasionally. Like if we've been working hard on something, she'll say 'I need a chocolate muffin!' And she'll eat it. Or she'll say 'Let's go to a restaurant. We deserve a good dessert.' She eats emotionally sometimes, but on a very small scale. Mostly she listens to her body.*

Along with shame, guilt has one of the lowest low scores on Dr Hawkins' Map of Consciousness. When chocolate, cake or malva pudding are as psychologically legal (note: I didn't say biologically legal) as carrots or broccoli, then the playing fields are equalled so that a person's choices are body- rather than deprivation-driven. Because non-Dietonians don't make a big issue about eating foods Dietonians feel guilt-stricken about, they don't feel the same deprivation followed by cravings and guilt-ridden-binges.

How to legalize food:
Buy a large enough of whatever food (let's say chocolate) it is that you consider to be illegal (and in as many varieties as you like). Buy enough so that you couldn't possibly eat it all in one sitting. Surround yourself with it: make sure it's in your home, at your place of work and readily available in a food bag. Then follow three simple rules:
The very next time that you really want to eat chocolate:
- ♥ Eat chocolate BUT ONLY chocolate for as long as it takes for your body to ask for something different. Chocolate for breakfast, lunch and supper.
- ♥ Savor each mouthful and take note of the tastes and textures
- ♥ Make a note of how your body feels immediately when you've eaten, 30 minutes later and a few hours later. Listen beyond the initial pleasure of unrestricted eating and hear what your body is telling you.

Even if you think you've died and gone to chocolate heaven, these feelings won't last for long... so. Promise! Before too long, your body will tell you what it wants – and don't be surprised if it's the first time in your life that you've ever craved a salad or wholesome veggie soup! Don't throw whatever chocolate left away, leave it surrounding you until it demands to be eaten again and then follow exactly the same rules as before. Keep doing this until you notice that your mind really doesn't seem that pre-occupied with eating chocolate anymore. Of course, you maybe have to now legalize something else and then something else until eventually you've convinced yourself that all foods really are legal.

A body pilgrim who tried the approach outlined above said: *It does really work. I always called myself a chocaholic, but now I realize it was just because it was considered an illegal food! Now I just don't have a burning desire to rush out and get tons of it and gobble it up in a panic! The trick is to constantly remind myself that all food is equal.*

Making sure you have sufficient quantities helps, because it allows you to reassure yourself that you won't be deprived. *I bought four slabs of Lindt chocolate. I hid them in my cupboard. The first two days I ate three slabs, and being afraid to run out I went to buy another two. The rule I had was that I would close my door, savor every mouthful, and not stop before I physically wanted to, even if it meant eating all four slabs. The first day I ate three slabs, the second day one. Then I didn't want it anymore. Now I have two and a half slabs left in my cupboard. I know it's there if I want it."*

Yes, I know, it really does sound like the strangest cure! And I'll admit it sure does turn the traditional 'knowledge' inside out, but it's an amazing way of letting your body know you are really going to trust it. So, let's say you've been avoiding bread. Mentally put bread on your 'allowed to eat' list and once your mind is satisfied that it is psychologically legal; you'll find you can enjoy bread without overeating it.

Legalizing is a process that happens in stages and it happens differently for each Dietonian. Some Dietonians are filled with sheer panic at the mere thought of allowing themselves this kind of freedom. *Having so much chocolate makes me paralysed. I'm paralysed with fear, paralysed with nausea, and feeling tired and just terrible.*

Some people feel like they'll get stuck right there, but eventually work through their fear. *I'm not one of those people who found legalizing a freeing process – it just felt terrifying. Then the worse possible thing happened (or so I thought). I started working at a pharmacy where they had candy and chocolate bars for sale. This was my nemesis, but also my legalizer... After four months of eating candy and chocolates almost every day, there wasn't a single candy or chocolate they sold that I wanted anymore.*

Other people get impatient because in our world of instant fixes, staying with the process of legalizing (which can take a while) is difficult when you don't see immediate measurable results. Then you grow doubtful about the process as this starting-out Dietonian says: *I say it's 'legalized and then I eat sugar because I'm feeling awful. I know I'm eating because of my emotions and then saying to myself that it's okay because I know what I'm doing. Of course I'm not changing my behaviour in the slightest.*

It's important for me to say, it rarely happens that we attempt legalizing and, instantly, it's a done deal! It takes time and frustration before you see the victory. Again, try to think of it being for the long-term good.

Some Dietonians leap in with gusto, experiencing an overwhelming feeling of liberation which is accompanied by making up for all the past deprivations. *At first I found myself bingeing on everything I'd never allowed myself to eat. It made me panic until I realized that the reason I was bingeing wasn't because I had legalized food, but rather because I was making up for all the previous deprivation of this food. After a while my body got tired of all the junk I was feeding it and started asking for more nutritious foods. It's amazing what a difference it makes to trust my body to tell me what it wants rather than having a dictatorial eating plan I have to stick to.*

For those like me, who have a tendency to buck against the feeling of being controlled, legalizing can become a great way to rebel. *Recently, since 'legalizing' all food, I've got into a habit of buying myself candy after work. Then I realized that I have not really legalized all food – all I have done is allow the rebel inside me to run free, getting high on sugar.* This is a vital connection to make. Rebelling isn't the same as legalizing! But we may first have to rebel (just to bring the scales of deprivation back into balance) before we can start to properly legalize. It's like we've lived on one side of the imbalance for so long, that it *has* to swing to the other side and almost overcorrect before it can come back to a more balanced place somewhere in-between.

And for some groups of people, like diabetics, the psychological hooks are doubled: *I've gone from health-obsessive to health-evasive. I've been trying to live like someone who is not diabetic. For me, ignoring high blood glucose levels is not self-loving. I know that. But I've been rebelling!* It is a problem getting stuck in that rebelling mode, not realizing that that is where you are instead of that place of legalizing. You should be aware that the giddy feeling of freedom and elation of rebelling are only 'superficial' legalizing. To truly legalize food and eating at a deep level, you need to move beyond these stages. At a real legalizing level, you are infused with a sense of calm and peacefulness, and the changes you make in your behaviour become sustainably effortless. It's the point at which your eating normalises – not because you're 'being good' but because you are no longer psychologically hooked into food. That is when you have truly legalized food.

SELF-LOVE IS EATING WITH CHILDLIKE CURIOSITY

Getting baby to eat as fast as possible is almost a prerequisite for busy parents in the modern frenetic lifestyle where we are constantly rushing from pillar to post. This emphasis on eating as much as possible in as short a time as possible becomes conditioned. *I grew up under constant threat of someone eating my food if I didn't shovel it in. My mother had a quick temper and often my food would get whisked into the dog's bowl because I was such a slow eater. As an adult, even if Mom isn't there, as soon as I'm around food I feel frantic to get to it as soon as possible.*

Carl Honore of the book *In Praise of Slow* encourages us to become a member of the Slow Food movement. This new cultural move towards living a slower-paced life has attracted over 78 000 members in more than 50 countries. From an eating perspective, slow eating is designed to combat the 'gobble-up-and-go' syndrome such as that found in fast-food places which pride themselves on their speed of service. Instead of spending the average 11 minutes to eat at McDonalds, slow restaurants encourage people to eat with family and friends in a much slower and more leisurely way.

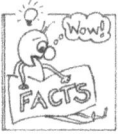

> When normal-weight college-age women consumed a large bowl of pasta they were first asked to eat the food quickly (they consumed 646 calories in nine minutes). On another occasion they were asked to eat the same meal but to really take their time (they consumed 579 calories in 29 minutes). When they ate quickly, the women were less satisfied and felt hungrier after completing the meal and for an hour afterwards compared to when they ate slowly. When they ate slower they reported really tasting their food and enjoying it more. [34]

One escaping Dietonian explained it: *Food tastes so much better when I'm actually hungry. As I get fuller, it's like my body doesn't taste it in the same way. This is a means of telling me that I need to think about stopping.*

Dr Ellen Langer, psychology professor at Harvard and author of *Mindfulness*, points out that it's a human tendency to operate on autopilot, performing mechanically or by rote or simply not paying attention. Few of us realize the extent to which we live mindlessly. *I don't think when I eat; it's like I don't want to. It's hand-to-mouth motion.* In contrast, Dr Langer defines 'mindfulness' as a way of thinking that focuses on taking in information with a degree of uncertainty and taking notice of new things.

In December of 2006, a new kind of 'dark' restaurant opened in Beijing. The lights are switched off and waiters serve food wearing special night goggles. Without being able to see their food, patrons savor the smell, texture and taste in more detail. This is a new experience in mindful eating. Eating (and even food preparation) can be beautifully mindful.

Self♥ = learning how to enjoy and savor food

When we have the mentality of a Dietonian we're inclined to feel helpless about our apparent love for food and to wish we didn't like eating as much as we do. With a Nature's Valley mentality, our aim is to get to know which foods we really do enjoy, and then to legalize our enjoyment of them. *I still love food and delicacies – the only difference now is that I savor and think about whatever I eat. My biggest achievement to date is not to devour food but to linger over the tastes. I must admit I enjoy my food even more now.*

The fascinating thing is that while we still think that certain foods are illegal, we don't really even taste them, but at the same time we're convinced we can't do without them. Legalizing eating and savoring the taste often means you discover that foods you once thought were delicious actually aren't! *I have just put my choccie muffin cravings to a rest! I have been having one whenever I felt like it. I ate slowly and enjoyed it – or rather tried to – but have now finally realized that I don't like them anymore. I don't know if I ever did. I just know that I won't want to eat them again. All this happened because they were legal and I could eat them when I wanted to.* I can't say this enough: legalizing is the way to removing that 'shimmer' that food has for us. *I had a thing for pecan nut pie. There is a coffee shop that made the most wonderful pecan nut pie. So every time I went to town, I would have it with ice cream. The last two times I did away with the ice cream. Yesterday I was the only one in the coffee shop. I ate my pecan nut pie with all my senses. I picked it with my fingers, smelt it, rubbed the crust between my fingers and savored every mouthful. Halfway, I didn't like it anymore. I left it, paid my bill and went to the restaurant next door for a chicken salad. That was what my body wanted.*

Mindfulness relies on a healthy respect for uncertainty and curiosity. They allow you to become more open-minded to re-experiencing the sensual pleasures of food. When you do re-examine the physical properties of food with open-minded mindfulness, you experience it in vastly different ways compared with when you eat as if you already know what to expect.

Do the The Joy-Filled Body taste test by mentally pretending to arrive on planet earth with no previous knowledge of any food. Adopt an attitude of curiosity and discovery and prepare yourself a 'taste-plate.' I suggest you try the following combination (but you're also welcome to make up your own): Take any kind of cheese and cut 4 small slices of it. Cut four slices of any dried fruit as well as its fresh equivalent (e.g. sultanas and grapes, prune and plums, dried peach/apple and fresh peach/apple) into approximately the same sizes as your slices of cheese.

♥ First mentally rate how much you like them on a scale of 1-10.
1 = this is disgusting, 5 = this is Ok, and 10 = this is orgasmically delicious.
Once you've rated your anticipated liking for each individual item take one at a time and:
   ♥ Look at it as if you have never seen it before. What do you notice about its color and appearance?
   ♥ Rub it between your fingers, How does it feel?
   ♥ Rub it on your lip. Does its texture change?

146

- ♥ Smell it. What happens in your mouth?
- ♥ Without biting it, move it around inside your mouth. Do you detect any flavor?
- ♥ Take a single bite, suck it and move it around your mouth. What do you notice?
- ♥ Close your eyes and chew on it, extracting maximum flavor for as long as possible.
- ♥ Notice the aftertaste. Do you like it? What else do you notice about the food in your mouth?
- ♥ Now re-rate. What do you notice – do you like it or dislike it as much as you thought you did?
- ♥ Then extend your taste test using various combinations: e.g. first do the above with a piece of cheese, then with the fresh fruit and then the dried fruit. Then swap the order – eat the dried fruit first then the fresh fruit and then the cheese. What do you notice about how the flavors and your liking of them change? Then try the cheese with a piece of the fresh fruit and compare it to cheese with the dried fruit? Which do you prefer and why?

Record what you noticed about this taste-test. What does this taste test tell you about how:

- ♥ you normally taste food
- ♥ what you discovered that possibly surprised or disappointed you?

When you're tasting and rating your food, you begin to make interesting discoveries about your eating. It's common for escaping Dietonians to be surprised at foods they discover they don't like.

I always thought I had to eat whatever food was given to me. But when I started rating my food on a scale of 1–10 in terms of whether I liked it or not, I realized I was eating a lot of things I didn't really like. So when food falls below a 5 rating on the delicious scale, I ask myself what that food is doing in my mouth. I'm worth eating food I really like.

Eating with childlike curiosity made me realize how much of my food I never even tasted. It was a case of gobble and gone! I found a new childlike delight in discovering what various foods felt like, smelt like and tasted like. Discovering some unhealthy food I didn't like was a revelation; I always thought there wasn't a food in the world I wouldn't find totally delicious.

When I went down for lunch today, I saw that they had made my favorite – chocolate mousse! I ate one spoonful of mousse and it was terrible! It felt fatty on my palate, so I took another mouthful just to make sure, but it was still awful. This is definitely a first for me!

It is a total revelation once escaping Dietonians start to realize that their old 'favorites' aren't quite what they always thought they were. They literally feel as if some amazing miracle has occurred. It is simply getting rid of the psychological blocks by getting your mind to gain fresh perspectives. It is MIND over Fatter!

Some practical morsel strategies to help you savor your food

I take an ordinary rubber band and wear it to act as a visual reminder that I'm trying to change unhelpful habits. It reminds me to stop and ask my body what hunger I'm experiencing or to eat slower. But it also has the additional advantage of, if I'm 'zoning out', I can just snap it on my skin, which immediately brings me back into the present moment.

I can't tell you how difficult it was for me to remember to slow down my eating. While I was chewing one mouthful, I was already loading up my fork with the next mouthful. While still chewing, I'd already be putting more food in. What worked for me was to put a yellow card in front of my plate with a big 'PUT DOWN' written on it in red letters. I couldn't help seeing it and it reminded me to put down my utensils between every mouthful.

I started to compete silently with everyone else at the table – I 'won' when I was the last person to finish eating. It gave me a secret kick to play this silly secret game. It also slowed down my eating and helped me to eat a lot less."

I always said I ate because I loved the taste of food. What made a difference for me was when someone pointed out that I only have taste buds on my tongue: as soon as I swallowed the food, the flavor was gone. This meant that if I loved the taste of something, I didn't need more of it, I needed to keep that same food on my tongue for longer. This way I eat less but enjoy food more."

SELF-LOVE IS CHOOSING BODY-FOOD

We're so strung up about *what* to eat, but no-one ever contemplates that there may be another really important factor to take into account. Is it possible that *what* you eat only really makes a real difference when you're flooding your body with the right life-supporting internal chemicals that are caused by high-energy attractor patterns of thought? Consider the following. In *What the*

Bleep do we know? Dr Candace Pert says, 'Our mind literally creates our body,' then she goes on to explain that the nature of receptors is that they change depending on what is happening to them.

So, if they are being bombarded by an internal chemical for a long time at a high intensity, they will shrink, or there will be fewer of them, or they become desensitised and need much more of the same internal chemical to achieve the original response. Dr Joe Dispensa, picking up on this knowledge, asks a thought-provoking question: 'If we're bombarding the same cell with the same attitude and the same chemistry over and over again – and on a daily basis – when that cell finally decides to divide…that new cell will have more receptor sites for those particular emotional neuropeptides and fewer receptor sites for vitamins, minerals, nutrients, fluid exchange or even the release of waste products or toxins.' So the question arises, Does it really matter what we eat? Does nutrition really have an effect if the cell, after 20 years of emotional abuse, doesn't *have* the receptor sites to receive or let in the nutrients necessary for its health? This is quite a mind-boggling thought because what he's saying is that *your unloving thoughts may be physically affecting your body's ability to utilise vitamins and minerals, despite you eating the healthiest possible foods!* That sure puts a new spin on the value of stemming the neuropeptide rush of life-eroding thoughts in favour of having life-supporting, self-loving ones.

Body-foods are those foods that your *body*, not your *mind* wants. It's the food your body chooses naturally once all the psychological hooks have been removed. They satisfy you.

We went out for dinner to Ocean Basket and instead of ordering my usual grilled fish, no butter and side salad I ordered the calamari and rice. I felt sooo satisfied. I didn't grab a mint or go home feeling like I wanted more, more, more...

It's not just about *knowing* what you want; it's about *having* what you want. Often you know exactly what you want – but you don't make a satisfactory plan to eat it. If you don't give your body what *it* wants and needs, everything else is wasted food.

I'm too impatient. I feel like something specific to eat, but can't wait long enough or take the time to find out, so I land up stuffing myself with something, anything, just to get food in.

How do you know which are body-foods?
Stop before you want to eat and ask your body these three questions:
♥ What Temperature food does my body feel like (hot or cold)?
♥ What Texture food does my body want (rough, smooth, liquid, solid)?
♥ What Taste do I feel like (savory, sweet, fishy, meaty, vegetable)?

NB: body-foods aren't ALWAYS only healthy choices, but they will be the vast majority of the time.

To help their bodies make healthy decisions, some escaping Dietonians make their food choice and then do one more body check, using visualisation.

I find it helpful to ask my body what it wants to eat and then to take just a second or two to imagine how this food might make my body feel as it becomes distributed into my cells. This way, if I 'saw' that eating a particular food was going to leave my veins feeling clogged up, and then I could choose a different food that wouldn't do that.

When you're a Dietonian, you become used to living a life of tricking yourself. You learn how to look at the food scale from an angle that allows you to eat more, you 'forget' the calories you consumed when you licked your son's ice-cream bowl clean. But with The Joy-Filled Body, there is no reason for tricking yourself because there is no deprivation and nothing is illegal. You can be completely honest and reasonable with your mind and body, as this body pilgrim discovered:

I loved asking my body what food it really wanted. My problem was that I always came up with something that I had to get into my car and drive to fetch, or something that was unobtainable. It was my way of saying, 'You see, this is a stupid idea, it won't work.' Eventually I realized I was putting obstacles in my own way. I started asking myself if I wanted something hot or cold, sweet or savory, then finding something available in that category, and offering that to myself.

Maybe you could also learn from other cultures – like the Italians, Indians and Chinese – who serve a variety of foods on the table all at once. Everyone can have a little of everything on the table and get to enjoy the different flavors. You're not restricted or deprived; you don't envy another's food or feel self-conscious about what is on your plate. Eating this way, you find that you are actually drawn to eating the things your body really wants, and despite the large amount of food on the table, you're also less likely to overeat because you're getting a variety of tastes.

Self♥ = believing you deserve good quality food

I've become more discerning. I enjoy and I appreciate food more, so I'm not going to eat rubbish or something that doesn't taste great.

In order for you, too, to become more discerning, eat the best that's available in your food choices – you deserve to! So if you're going to eat chocolate, eat the product or label you like most of all, then savor it.

I can no longer eat normal cheap chocolate. I either buy quality chocolate or no chocolate at all – and I eat one block at a time.

Choosing the more expensive chocolate over cheaper, plastic-tasting ones and really savoring it is actually an action of self-love. It is not nurturing to gobble down something you don't even like that much.

Next, don't eat a salad when you really want chocolate because it won't satisfy that need. And ultimately you'll still crave the chocolate you never allowed yourself, so you'll eat it on top of everything else – because that's what you really wanted. *I sometimes have pudding as dinner. I feel a lot better doing that because before I'd force myself to eat a healthy meal (when I wasn't hungry) so that I would have the 'right' to the sweet stuff afterwards. Surprise, surprise – I gained weight! Now I eat only sweet stuff if that's what I feel like.*

Even if you know it possibly isn't your healthiest choice, don't eat guiltily. Without all the guilt and self-chastisement, your body will simply self-correct and choose healthier food later.

As I've said earlier, body-foods aren't always healthy foods, but your body appears to have an intrinsic knowledge of and preference for healthy foods.

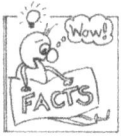

For example, an audience that did not know the difference between two similar-looking apples universally went weak during muscle testing when shown an apple grown with pesticides but stayed strong when the apple was organic. And when Dr Hawkins handed out identical envelopes containing either organic vitamin C or artificial sweeter, all of the 1000-strong audience, who had no knowledge of the contents of the envelopes, gave a weak muscle response to the artificial sweetener and a strong muscle response to the vitamin C. There is a universal intelligence our bodies have about food that we cannot always easily explain. [35]

SELF-LOVE IS OVERCOMING OVEREATING

Self♥ = not sentencing yourself to a punishing regime

Prescriptive diets where you unnaturally disrupt your life, or put it on hold, can only ever be temporary. I'm reminded of the BBC1 'Diet Trials' TV series where the judge looks down his nose, taps his gavel and says sternly, 'You have been sentenced to six months of a dietary regime.' And that's the problem! Anything that you feel 'sentenced' to doing for however long (not that many of the diet trialists lasted six months, by the way) is simply not a plan for life. To reach Nature's Valley, you need to make changes that are sustainable forever. Anything you start that has you feeling as if you've been sentenced to a life of restriction and deprivation is doomed to fail… the only variable is how long it takes.

Self♥ = doing whatever it takes to eat whenever you're physically hungry

Your cells are working to save your life, so each time you deprive them they slow your metabolism and increase your appetite so that you eat more. Tabitha Hume, author of The X-diet, likens the way your muscles digest food to an army. If you start depriving your body of carbs that is, depriving your muscle 'army' of its fuel, then the army is faced with a crisis and turns on itself. It starts to eat up itself as fuel, and you lose muscle mass. This shows as a weight loss, because muscle weighs more than fat. The biggest problem happens when you start eating carbohydrates again. Your cells assume you have just survived a famine. Because your muscle army is now vastly reduced, it can't consume all this food, and being the helpful little things they are, your cells store any excess food you eat as fat so you'll be ready for the next 'famine'.

It's important to eat for biological reasons, but more importantly, it prevents the feelings of deprivation that lead to all kinds of sneak-eating. *At about six at night everybody is starting to look for something to eat, but my mom is tired and tells everybody she's not the only person responsible for preparing food. But, if someone else starts doing something about supper, my mom goes on this guilt trip and tells us that she knows she is a bad mom, which leads to a very uncomfortable situation and nobody eating! Later, everybody starts sneaking into the kitchen to try to find something to eat without anybody seeing them. All of us have a problem with eating late at night.*

Don't allow someone else's problem to become your reason for sneak-eating. When someone lays a guilt trip on you this in this way, try to see it for what it is – an opportunity to change an old unhelpful pattern.

Self♥ = banishing 'last chance' eating

Frantic eating often has to do with 'the last supper' kind of scenario in which you eat as a way of staving off anticipated future deprivation. *People often eat pizza or a chocolate 'for the last time' before they start their diet… I'm eating this for the last time – that's why I'm eating it so fast.*

'Last chance' eating has an attitude of 'eat as much as you can', which you develop when trapped in Diet City – next time you see food like this you won't be allowed to eat it because of the diet you're on. Fears of not getting your share or not getting the best part of a particular food are all psychological hooks that keep you eating as if it's your last chance. *At family functions there is always too much food, sometimes the best things go first, and then you feel like, Damn, I should've eaten some when I had the chance.*

I have two oatmeal cookies because they are delicious and I really feel like them. Then I stop and think to ask myself, do I really need another one? Sometimes, illogical as it is, I see that cookie jar hopping around in the cupboard screaming, 'I'm going to leave if you don't eat these cookies now!' I have to tell myself, Tomorrow is another day, and I can have some more tomorrow.

Self♥ = reminding yourself there's enough food in your world

Few Dietonians in our Western culture are reacting to a realistic fear of there not being enough food. It's those conditioned psychological hooks that are getting to us. *I have two brothers and when they were teenagers, man, oh man, the way they ate! It reached a stage where I would eat something even if I wasn't hungry or in the mood, because I just knew that later there would be none left (especially party-type foods)."* Now I have this anxiety about things being sold out – like what if I get to the shop/bakery and my favorite foods are sold out (it has happened), so I guess I have this mentality of 'better get it while I can'.

Isn't it strange, though, that we don't seem to have the same anxieties around healthy foods not being there for us? It is only the foods that we've been conditioned to think of as 'treat' food, or 'reward' food, or 'this'll make you feel better' food that we fear becoming unavailable. *Of course I don't feel this way about stuff like bread or carrots - just stuff like chocolate cheesecake and lasagne. I mean, I'm really embarrassed to admit this, but I've even been known to wake up in the middle of the night to eat the last of something with glee – feeling childlishly happy that I got the last of the good stuff.*

Self♥ = protecting yourself from feelings of deprivation

We can also have a sense of deprivation that has resulted from having to share or compete for food. *My mom would tell me to hide my diet/special food in my room so that my brother couldn't get it.*

I used to get so fed up when I baked or bought a cake or a tart, because being the only female amongst three males, I was lucky to get one piece of anything before it was finished. So I divided everything in four equal pieces or amounts – that way they could eat theirs in one go if they wanted to, but mine would last because I prefer to eat a smaller piece every day.

When I stocked up on illegal foods (cookies, jerky, chocolate), was so afraid my family would get hold of them that I gobbled them up the first chance I got. Now I hide my food. It's amazing how long the packet seems to be lasting these days! I eat them whenever I want them – depriving myself is counterproductive.

Most people might think hiding food is a sign that something is seriously wrong – but this is not the same as sneak-eating and in the context of legalizing food, it can be a self-loving action to protect your food source in this way. Remember the context: feelings of deprivation create psychological hooks, which you want to get rid of.

Self♥ = leaving food (even when you've paid for it)

Many Dietonians grew up hearing 'waste not, want not' and find it difficult not to clean their plates. *I was so used to finishing my baby's left-over Purity – it was a habit fuelled by all those stories of starving children when I was a child. Eventually I stuck a note on her feeding tray to remind myself that my body wasn't a dumpsite.* What you are *not* doing here is listening to your body (unless, of course, you are eating because you're physically hungry at this particular time), but you also don't want to become a role-model for your children to imitate.

Once all foods are legal for you and you also have legalized leaving food on the plate, it will surprise you how you're able to go anywhere and survive being faced with any foods. *I was at the movies with my cousin and afterwards we went to Milky Lane for ice-cream. Her sundae had cream on top of it, but she didn't really like the taste of it. Her husband told her to mix it in with the ice-cream so the taste wouldn't be so bad. She said, 'No.' The Mind over Fatter principle is that you don't eat things you don't like the taste of. Classic! So she scraped the cream off. Her sundae also had Cadbury's Whispers on it, which she also took off. In the days before Mind over Fatter I'd have eaten the Whispers so as not to waste them. But I didn't want them, so I didn't.*

Restaurants and other places where we have paid for the food are challenging to us, because as Dietonians, we have to overcome the inclination to 'get our money's worth'. *Economists have a theory about 'sunk costs' and it can be applied to buying food in a restaurant. Whether you eat the food you have ordered or not, you're going to pay for it. It's a sunk cost, you can write it off! Eating something you don't like just because you paid for it makes things worse, because you're paying for it 'twice'. If that cake is on the dry side, why should you pay for it: first in cash, then in feelings of guilt (not for eating cake, but for consuming unsatisfying calories)!*

SELF-LOVE IS STOPPING WHEN YOU'VE HAD ENOUGH

Not only should you leave food that is not to your taste, but you should also leave food that you know is going to leave you feeling overfull. *Yesterday I bought two pies, but after the first pie I already felt full. However I insisted on trying to eat the second pie. Less than halfway through I had to admit that I couldn't, not because I'm a hero, but simply because I really was no longer hungry.* Soon you'll register how good your body feels when you stop eating in time. *I looked at those last few mouthfuls of food and had a moment of clarity: my body felt good right now; it didn't need another morsel more. In that moment, I knew I really liked that feeling of not having over-eaten.*

The best way to move from eating for plate-size to eating for tummy-size is making choices that fuel your 'want' power to do what makes you and you body feel good. *I was just about to take a habitual mouthful of the roast potato that I really wanted to leave because I was already full. I remembered that eating that potato might be the easy choice, but it really wasn't the self-loving choice. That made it much easier to toss it because as much as I love roast potatoes, I really do want to be more loving towards myself.*

Self♥ = not eating to satisfy others' needs

For many Dietonians, plate-cleaning is quite often an emotionally-charged event with many psychological hooks. *My mother was a single parent and had to carry two to three jobs so that we could have food on the table. To make up for the time she wasn't around she used to make huge meals with loads of comfort-foods and expected us to eat every little bit. She would take huge exception if you didn't clean your plate!*

In our culture, the preparation of food is often a way of showing love, thus rejecting food is tantamount to rejecting someone's love. *My mother-in-law is obsessed with feeding people and she measures people's response to her in how much they enjoy her food. If you don't eat her food you don't like her, or there is something wrong with you!* Lots of eating is done in the name of not wanting to hurt the feelings of another. But it's a brave step to realize that not hurting *yourself* should be your first priority. *I'm at the point where, if I'm at a party and I put food on my plate only to discover later that I don't like the taste of some of the food, I'm simply not going to eat it. Now some people (especially my mother's generation) might think I'm rude but, hey, that's your issue, not mine.*

SELF-LOVE IS BEATING SNEAK-EATING

During one online conversation on the Mind over Fatter forum about sneak-eating, someone asked: *Why do we feel so embarrassed to say what we eat?* The answer she received was very insightful: *I think that this is just another hangover from Diet City, from feeling we'll be 'judged' and 'found guilty' by the diet-police. We don't feel embarrassed if the food we are eating is accepted as 'diet food.* People who have never been caught in Diet City can't even begin to imagine that someone feels ashamed about being seen eating – to them it's a foreign concept. But it's very real for Dietonians. *It took me a looong time before I felt able to eat in the open. I have a big basket of food that I take to work everyday. I imagine everyone's looking at me, shaking their heads and thinking, well, that's why she's so fat... I have had to remind myself that what I am doing is good self-care. If I don't feed my tummy when it asks for food, then I am going to have trouble later.* And she's absolutely right – you need to fuel your body at the time it genuinely needs food. And you need to feed it every time it let's you know it's hungry and regardless of what others might think. This is honouring your body's needs and feeding it well prevents feelings of deprivation.

Self ♥ = no longer guiltily sneak-eating

When we go camping at the end of the year, my hubby buys all the candy I love. Who sneaks back to the caravan to gobble some marshmallows? ME. When he asks where all the candy has gone, I tell him it's the monkeys (this monkey, yes!). Once I've emptied the packet I regret what I've done and then sulk or moan about my fat ass! Secretive eating means we eat as quickly as we can and as much as we can for fear of being caught out. If you were a naturally slender person you'd be able to eat everything on the list without feeling you had to hide it simply because it would be legal to eat it. If you were legalizing all the candy you love, this kind of sneak-eating wouldn't be a part of your life. Sneak-eating is *always* a signal that there is something you needs to legalize.

If you're feeling tempted to sneak-eat ask yourself these questions:
What have I not yet legalized?
♥ is it this specific food?
♥ is it eating in front of this particular person?
♥ is it legalizing eating this kind of food in public?
♥ is it that eating even for the overweight is a necessity?

SELF-LOVE IS REMAINING CALM AROUND FOOD

Self ♥ = enjoying food guiltlessly

Dietonians (especially if you think of yourself as fat) convince themselves that to enjoy or be seen to enjoy eating is a criminal act. Your mind becomes so hooked into monitoring what, when and how you eat that when you get to eat in public, it feels like you're in a minefield. *A social event involving eating is like a mountain for me to climb. The energy it takes to tell myself, No, you've had enough, No, you don't need it, NO this, NO that . . . it's such a mental challenge that I am actually exhausted afterwards.*

When you're a resident of Nature's Valley, the 'no's' don't exist because the 'can't haves' weren't there in the first place. It's also easy to feel quite daunted at the thought of taking your time to savor and enjoy your food lest other people see you still busy EATING! *At the moment I don't feel comfortable enjoying food – I just want to get it out of the way. I've also noticed when I'm around food I have this rushed feeling as if something is chasing me.* It's a sad fact that eating at a leisurely pace isn't a problem for people who don't have issues with eating, but for those of us who do, it can feel enormous. Feelings of self-consciousness and being judged by others are prevalent. *I'm very self-conscious about being the last one still eating – it makes me feel as if everyone is staring at me, sniggering and telling each other it's no wonder I'm fat because all they ever see me doing is eating. It makes me want to eat as much as possible as quickly as possible.*

Those escaping from Diet City need to keep on reminding themselves that eating is an essential part of a healthy and wholesome life. They are as deserving as the next person when it comes to enjoying their food. It takes courage to persevere, but take a few deep breaths and silently repeat the words, 'Be calm, eating is essential'. If you keep on listening to your body and make choices that are right for it, you *will* get through this.

Slowing down and eating mindfully are ways Dietonians will find helpful to get themselves to stay calm around food. *At times I find myself eating in an uncontrollable way. I used to do that often and then stick my finger down my throat, but I always felt awful about myself. Now I've taught myself to push my plate away or get up from the table and just take a few breaths until I feel calm in front of food again.*

After I've dropped the kids at school and been to the gym, it feels so peaceful to sit quietly and take 15 minutes out of my hectic day to enjoy my breakfast. I like to put on some soothing music because eating in this way sets the tone for the rest of my day and I feel more relaxed and find stresses easier to deal with without resorting to food. On days when I'm extra rushed, I remind myself that 15 minutes isn't going to rob me of time because of the added calm it always gives me.

I was forever eating on the wing. It may seem stupid, but I needed to remind myself I wasn't committing a crime if I took 20 minutes to sit and eat quietly. I find such pleasure in the simple act of eating, chewing and really tasting.

I told myself if I wasn't getting enough of love from others, it was my responsibility to give it to myself because when I felt loved, I was a better wife, mother and friend. Now I think of eating as taking a self-love pill – only it takes 20 minutes or so to swallow.

Self♥ = handling binges differently

Geneen Roth, well-known writer on weight issues, says that a binge isn't dependent on the amount of food you eat or what you eat but by the *way* you eat it. A cup of ice-cream can be a binge if you eat it with an urgent franticness and a desperate need to zone out. It's the same as the drug addict desperately needing to get into an altered state. *There are definitely parallels in the desperation that a drug addict and a binge eater feel. I'm talking mad desperation here, and I'm pretty sure that many of us have been there – that feeling of spiralling out of control and being helpless to stop it, not even sure whether you want to stop it...*

A binge is a signal that something is badly wrong, that you are ignoring your needs – either physically (by eating low quantities or low-quality foods) or emotionally (a need for connection, love companionship). Binges are often your response to physical or emotional deprivation; they're a way of finally giving to yourself without holding back.

The next time you want to binge, tell yourself that you can and will take one minute - to be with yourself before you eat. Wanting to binge is a reminder to stop, step back and take some time for you. Promise yourself that much time to do nothing before you start eating. Respond to your body's call to get your attention. Sit down, breathe a few times, and with as much curiosity as you can muster, gently ask yourself:

- ♥ What do you need?
- ♥ Who do you need it from?
- ♥ What would be the kindest thing you could do for yourself now?
- ♥ What would happen if you didn't eat? (Would you *really* throttle your boyfriend/child/ mother/sister or kick the dog? Remember that doing what you think you want to and actually doing it are two different things.)
- ♥ What if you allowed yourself to just observe yourself having the full range of your feelings without judging them, or fearing that having these feelings means acting on them?
- ♥ What if instead of eating, you curled up on your bed or couch with a soft blanket? Did nothing for a while?
- ♥ What if you gave yourself some kindness that didn't also hurt you at the same time?

What I have found helpful when this has happened to me is to try to NOT be frustrated with myself – rather to forgive myself and try to 'talk' to my body and find out more about it. For example, I would say, 'Okay, so you binged on sugar. You must have needed the comfort at this time. I'm not cross with you (my body). I will sit here now and try to work out why you needed to binge so that next time I won't subject you to this discomfort.' Remember that your body has intelligence: via the communication between your brain and your nervous system, it 'hears' your thoughts and reacts chemically to them. You can't actually separate your body and mind because it's your 'bodymind' (your emotional body) that knows the answers to the 'why' behind your behaviour.

For example, let's say you're bingeing and when you stop long enough to check-in with your body it brings to your attention that (for example) you seem to be trying to stuff down a lump in your throat. Ask yourself what's going on that you're feeling a symptom in that specific part of the body? In this case, our throat houses our vocal cords. If it feels as if your throat has a blockage - could it be that your body is trying to signal to you that you're feeling blocked about verbalizing something?

And then, let's be brutally realistic about what bingeing does for you in the long term. *I would think of whether the bingeing actually helped me in any way – did it comfort me? Did it make me feel empowered? Or did I feel sore and uncomfortable afterwards?*

To help you develop calmness around food, do this check list:

- ♥ If I eat now HOW am I feeling about eating: A frantic desperateness? A calmness?
- ♥ If I eat now WHAT kind of hunger will I be filling: Head? Throat? Heart? Or Tummy?
- ♥ If I eat my food of choice now, HOW will my body respond? Will it jump up and down with delight or feel sluggish and want to hide out?
- ♥ If I eat now HOW long do I have to eat? Will I savor and enjoy or be doing a grab 'n go number?
- ♥ If I eat now HOW will I know when my body feels satisfied?
- ♥ Once I've eaten, HOW will I remember to check in with my body as I stop eating, half an hour later and few hours later?

SELF-LOVE IS PRACTISING LOVING WAYS

Self♥ = acknowledging even the smallest steps

Realize that in trying to change a stubborn behaviour you will make the same mistakes several times over. It's often in walking down that street and falling into that same old hole a number of times, you realize you don't want to keep falling into it anymore. *I take so long to learn . . . I remember that I don't like the after-effect of things that are full of sugar. That brownie tasted very good, but not good enough that I'm prepared to endure the bad feeling that follows. I am still learning, though, to come to a standstill and think before I act.* Of course, having a realization like this doesn't mean we won't – and don't – fall back into the same hole again. It just means we've taken an important step towards cementing the fact that *we want to* stop falling into that hole. *I was surprised to realize that actually I was hungry and what I really wanted was food, not candy. It was a big moment. Habit prevailed though, and I opted for the marzipan choc log rather than jerky, but never mind, at least I'm taking baby steps.*

You may manage initially to avert the hole, but still land up falling into it afterwards – that is all part of the process, because so often, falling back into the hole provides us with an opportunity to discover something else. With ongoing awareness and consciously making new choices, you are eventually able to start walking around the hole without falling into it. *Last night I actually CHOSE to eat salad because that's what I really felt like. The down side is that I still ate candy afterwards – but I realized that in comparison, I didn't enjoy the taste!*

160

I decided that although cottage cheese does not taste the same, I am gonna try and substitute with it. I used to be addicted to toasted cheese sandwiches, but can't remember when last I had one.

When it comes to replacing one habit with another (remember those old established neural pathways), it can sometimes be really helpful to keep up the old habit alongside the new one for a while. So, instead of thinking, I'm scared to feel my emotions; I want to eat, move to: I want to eat but I know I'd like to feel a bit too, and that's okay. Then, after a while, you'll find it's easier to move on to, I want to feel, and I don't need to eat about it right now.

Self♥ = being awed by your accomplishments

With the growing awareness you gain, you can also start feeling awe for the progress you are making. *It's astonishing to see some of the food I bought, food over which I thought I had no control, laying for days in the kitchen, completely forgotten! And it is so real. And so freeing!* Feeling a sense of gratitude for your accomplishments is a high-energy attractor pattern. That sense of wonderment at a change you've made (no matter how small) builds hope because it confirms that change is possible without all those struggles involved in dieting. It confirms you're on the right road and it builds hope in your ability to make sustainable changes. *I often find myself in awe of the fact that I've managed to get to the stage in my life when food no longer controls me!*

Self♥ = getting helpful support

There is so much support out there for you – from trained professionals, people undergoing the same experience as you, even family and friends. Sometimes, it can be helpful to have the 'voice' of someone else to help us talk down the voice that urges us to eat. *My therapist said a very interesting thing to me: What's comforting and soothing is not necessarily good for you. Then last night I was planning a good old sugar binge but I just couldn't do it. Every time I thought about it, I heard his words. They were far too real for me to allow my usual self-deceit of 'I need it'.* Therapy might not be for everyone, but there are other means of support, like the free Mind over Fatter online group Mindoverfatter@yahoogroups.com. [35] These are typical posts from the site: *For many of us it's not about the food – it's about other issues. For me a big part of it was heart hunger and a bit of head hunger. But being able to talk about things and having the emotional support that this group gives me, I am no longer as dependent on food for comfort. I'm so thankful to have this group to support me on my journey.*

I am really overwhelmed with gratitude for all the love in this group. All the hope and encouragement, and all the honesty. We live in such a cynical word, but you guys make me believe in miracles. And if I didn't believe in God, you guys would make me believe that there is a God, a loving God, because I see evidence of this love in you. It's just amazing to me how a group of strangers can be drawn together in a common goal, through shared pain to help each other, and to celebrate each other's victories.

One body pilgrim had her husband read up on the legalizing process as a way of getting his support. He didn't judge her actions or pressurise her with comments like, 'This is such a dumb idea,' and instead was able to respect her choice and stand by her as she journeyed through the process. *When I drove up the driveway and saw my hubby in the garage I felt a bit tearful. He knows about this experiment because I encouraged him to read what you suggest so as not to give me added pressure by telling me I'm being ridiculous and make me feel even worse. When I saw him, l told him I was scared and this experiment is scary and not something I have done before. I asked him to please be patient with me.*

It's really important to communicate with those around you in ways that they understand what you're trying to achieve. Instead of trying to explain yourself (particularly since at first you may feel rather uncertain about things that seem so opposite to the traditional methods), select sections of this book and ask your loved one to read them. Better still, have them read the entire book as well as the Mind over Fatter program! And most important, if they ask you questions to which you don't have the answer, be honest and say so. But also e-mail us so we can help you. E.mail us at either : info@ditch-diets-live-light.com or info@mindoverfatter.co.za. Either way we'll be sure to get back to you. We want to be there to support and help you through the process.

SELF-LOVE IS COPING WITH SLIPS, DIPS AND DIVES

On this journey to Nature's Valley, it's not always easy to stay on a linear course. When you stray you have to depend on your attitude – your The Joy-Filled Body compass, if you like – to get you back on course. Very often, 'a slip becomes a dip and then turns into a dive.' But first it happens in your mind before it becomes a reality. Whether a small mistake becomes a dip or a dive depends on what you tell yourself.

Self♥ = not panicking at not getting the desired outcome

Be warned! Dedicated Dietonians are so used to being 'losing weight' focused and then having their diets fail them that they often start the The Joy-Filled Body journey wondering how long this 'diet' will last before they fall off the wagon once more. But this isn't another diet, this is a health-gain program and there is no such thing as failure. Every step to reclaiming your power to eat naturally produces an outcome – and this outcome is not right or wrong. It's just a natural result of your action. The Joy-Filled Body is not an A to B, as-the-crow-flies journey; it's more of an exploration. So if the step you take isn't producing the outcome you're looking for, don't panic! Simply make a mental note of what didn't work and take a different step. Keep doing this until you find an outcome you like. It's about making choices about which steps work for you and your life, instead of having them dictated to you.

Self♥ = seeing your mis-steps as potential to grow

It's not your missteps and stumblings that are problematic, it's when you become paralysed with fear or guilt about them, and you don't take the time to learn and grow through them. *I must admit that when I have been mad/sad/glad and needed to comfort-eat, NOTHING I do will take away that urge! Sometimes I just say to myself, okay self, so go and eat that chocolate – but make it count. Be fully aware of the moment, and forgive yourself. Then afterwards, I sit quietly and my self-talk goes like this: That chocolate was delicious, but what did I want it to do for me? And did it really do that?*

Self♥ = banishing black-and-white thinking

As I've mentioned previously, Dietonian thinking is often characterised by black-and-white thoughts: we're either 'good' or 'bad'; food is either 'legal' or 'illegal', and so on. This kind of thinking also confuses us about what qualifies as 'good enough' progress on the road to Nature's Valley. *I have been so bad – yesterday I ate a whole nougat bar and I feel so upset!* Eating a whole nougat bar isn't as terrible as the way this pilgrim is judging herself – and that's difficult for her to see. Just being aware that she ate it and she wished she hadn't is a step in the right direction and 'good enough' for the initial stages of her journey. When you label things as either 'wrong' or 'right', you're basically saying there is only one way of making the journey to Nature's Valley. That creates a lack of balance and disallows any room for growth and change. *I just don't think balance is something I have ever had!*

163

It's definitely been 'all or nothing' for EVERYTHING in my life! It's either right or wrong.

Somewhere in-between black and white are all the colours of the rainbow – and a few shades of grey too! Black-and-white thinking is only a set of principles you *believe* to be true, they have simply been ingrained into your neural pathways at the address where you grew up. They aren't Deep Truths; they're surface truths according to your specific culture. You need to learn to live with the full spectrum of colour.

Self♥ = banishing catastrophizing

Many Dietonians can attest to the effect that breaking even one dietary rule has on their ability to stick to whatever diet they are on. *The stricter the diet, the easier it is to slip up. I allowed room for not doing Mind over Fatter 100% correctly, and adopted the approach of being body-wise 80% of the time. Then when I wasn't body-wise, it wasn't a slip-up I had to punish myself for; it was just the 20% part of the equation. There was something about allowing myself to be less than perfect that allowed me to be much kinder to myself and kindness was much more effective than harsh self-judgement had ever been.*

Inflexible black-and-white thinking encourages catastrophizing – which *always* makes things worse. *It wasn't breaking some or other dietary rule that was really the problem; it was how harshly I judged my lack of willpower that made me really binge badly. I learnt that if I didn't catastrophize my slip-up, it didn't turn into an eating frenzy. So, when I ate something I wished I hadn't, I stopped myself from coming to conclusions of how awful, terrible and weak I was. That made it so much easier to get back on track. I found I stopped attacking everything in the fridge.* Catastrophizing leads Dietonians into that other trap – the what-the-heck-I've-blown-it-might-as-well-start-again-on-Monday syndrome. *I was so used to going on diet on a Monday, breaking it by the Thursday, and then spending the weekend eating frantically. Practically every Monday was the start of a new diet. On Mind over Fatter, all I had to do if I'd 'blown it' was to wait until I was hungry again before I ate. That was all – what a revelation!*

My passion for helping others liberate themselves from Diet City is driven by the memory I have, that when I was forever dieting, self-love was an impossible dream. Wonderful parts of me were dying. Parts of me were so taken up with obsessive monitoring of what I could and couldn't eat, what I had and hadn't eaten, that my life was narrow and shallow. I want you to live a life that is wide and deep. The Joy-Filled Body gives you the tools to *live* fully, joyously and without worries of food and eating.

Chapter 8

♥

Epilogue

Allowing your Essential and playful self to resurface and trusting your body to lead you there are seldom overnight events. Sadly, the fairy godmother and her wand have gone on holiday so this isn't an 'abracadabra' or 'open sesame' process that can be hurried along. We have to undo years of conditioning that have only succeeded in separating us from incredibly wise parts of our wonderful selves. The tiniest morsel in this book may have been the one that touched you deeply and helped you make profound new choices. And hopefully many of the bits of wisdom The Joy-Filled Body pilgrims have had the courage to share have awoken your own wisdom or helped you feel less alone with your problem. The morsels chosen were those that will help you the most to make moment-by-moment decisions that will lead to living a more harmonious and self-loving life. With growing your love of self and allowing yourself the freedom to play and trust yourself more comes health gain. Then weight loss will follow naturally, if that's what your body needs.

So, in a nutshell, here is the map to reaching Nature's Valley.

Allow all your decisions, day by day, meal by meal, activity by activity, to be guided by self-love. At each tiny crossroad, step back momentarily and do a mental check. Ask yourself:

Intuitively, what do I suspect this choice (food choice, choice of exercising, the attitude I'm adopting) is going to do for my body's biochemistry and how will that impact on the shape of my cellular crystals, my DNA telemores, my muscle strength and my immune system? Is this a love-based, health-enhancing choice or a fear and stress-based, health-eroding choice? Your body 'knows' what choices are good and bad for it – it's your mind that has become confused. This is why it's important to rely on the wisdom of your body.

And how will you know when you have finally escaped Diet City and arrived back at Nature's Valley? Simple! Food and eating will become a joy instead of something to fear. Your body will no longer be an enemy to monitor and watch with mistrust. Instead you'll find that body worries shrink and dissolve as you gain newfound respect for your body's ability to self-regulate. Sure there will be times when you overeat, comfort-eat, eat poor-quality food or make other non-self-loving choices – but instead of berating yourself, you'll simply notice it, and then let it go and move on.

There will probably be times when you pick up a few pounds, but instead of feeling desperate and worrying, I've got to diet, you'll think, That's interesting, I wonder what my body is trying to tell me? You'll be a lot more curious than judgemental, and you'll know that the work to be done isn't on your eating but on your emotional body. You'll use episodes like this to help you grow rather than to derail you. In fact, fad diets and adverts for all the diet paraphernalia will no longer interest you. Being active won't be a dreaded chore; it'll just feel like a natural part of living. You'll challenge culturally imposed surface truths and live more according to deep Creator-made truths. And you'll know that you're a fabulous Sacred Being, no matter what your size or shape.

P.S. (and you can blame me if this happens!) You may even be lucky enough to take yourself a lot less seriously and become much more in touch with that crazy, zany part of

References

Introduction

1. Schwartz, Vartanian, Nosek and Brownell. 'The Influence of One's Own Body Weight on Implicit and Explicit Anti-fat Bias' in *International Journal of Obesity* (2006).
2. Rodin, J, Silberstein, L & Striegel-Moore. 'Women and Weight: a Normative Discontent,' Yale University. In TB Sonderegger (Ed). 'Nebraska symposium on Motivation: Psychology and Gender', pp267–307, Lincoln: University of Nebraska Press.
3. Ibid.
4. Garner, DM, Wooley, SC. 'Confronting the Failure of Behavioral and Dietary Treatments for Obesity' in *Clinical Psychology Review*, Vol. 11, pp920–780, 991.
5. Leith, W. *The Hungry Years* (2005), p250, Bloomsbury.
6. Rodin, J, Silberstein, L and Striegel-Moore, ibid.
   6a. *Copenhagen Post* (20 Oct 2006)
   6b(http://news.independent.co.uk/health/article3138352.ece)
7. *Copenhagen Post*, 20 Oct 2006.
8. Dulloo, AG, Jacquet, J, and Montani, J-P. 'Pathways from Weight Fluctuations to Metabolic Diseases: Focus on Maladaptive Thermogenesis during Fat Catch-up' in *International Journal of Obesity* (2002), pp546–558.
9. Bacon, Linda, Stern, JS, van Loan, MD and Keim, NC. 'Size, Acceptance and Intuitive Eating helps Obese, Female, Chronic Dieters' in *Journal of the American Dietetic Association* (2005), pp105, 929–36.
10. Jorgensen, ME, Glumer, C, Bjerregaard, P, Gyntelberg, F, Jorgensen, T, Borch-Johnsen, K. 'Greenland Population Study' in *International Journal of Obesity 27* (2003), pp1507–15.
11. Andres, R. 'Effect of Obesity on Total Mortality' in *International Journal of Obesity 4*, pp 380–6 (1980).

12. Waaler, HT. 'Height, Weight and Mortality: the Norwegian Experience' in *Acta Med. Scandinavian Supplement 679* (1984), pp1–56.
13. Ernsberger, P. 'Is it Unhealthy to be Fat?' in *Radiance* (Winter 1986), p12.
14. Adapted from Maya Snijders-Naumann.

Ch. 2 Your Emotional Body

15. Hebb, Donald, *Organization of Behavior* (1949) (Canada). Out of print.
16. Pert, Dr Candace, Marriott, Nancy. *Everything you Need to Know to Feel Go(o)d*, p10, Hay House.
17. Hawkins, Dr David. *Power vs. Force*, Veritas. (See also www.veritaspub.com. Hawkins is a co-author with Nobel Prize winner Linus Pauling of *Orthomolecular Psychiatry*.)
18. Emoto, Dr Masaru. *The Secret Messages of Water*, Beyond Words Publishing. (See also www.masaru-emoto.net)
19. McCraty, Rollin; Atkinson, Mike; Rein, Glen; and Watkins, Alan D. 'Music Enhances the Effect of Positive Emotional States on Salivary IgA' in *Stress Medicine 12 (3)* (1996), pp167–175, and Rein, Glen; Atkinson, Mike; and McCraty, Rollin. 'The Physiological and Psychological Effects of Compassion and Anger' in *Journal of Advancement in Medicine 8 (2)* (1995), pp87–105.
20. Pert, Dr Candace, Marriott, Nancy. Ibid. See also *Molecules of Emotion by Dr Pert (Simon and Schuster),* and www.candacepert.com
21. McCraty, Rollin; Atkinson, Mike; Rein, Glen; and Watkins, Alan D. Ibid.
22. National Academy of Sciences, California (2004).
23. Khumalo, L. 1995. 'We like them Beefy' in *Drum* (December), pp114–116.
24. Khumalo, L. (ibid) and Sheward, D. 'Prevalence of Eating Disorders at Three Universities in the Western Cape,' unpublished Masters thesis (1994), University of Cape Town.
25. Wiseman, CV, Gray, JJ, Mosimann, JE, Ahrens, AH 'Cultural Expectations of Thinness in Women: an Update' in *International Journal of Eating Disorders*, Vol. 11 (1992), pp85–89.

Ch. 3 What's Eating Us

26. Swartz, L. 'Illness Negotiation: The Case of Eating Disorders' in *Social Sciences Medicine* Vol 24. No. 7 (1987), pp613–18.
27. National Sleep Foundation (USA). See www.sleepfoundation.org.
28. Sark. *Succulent Wild Woman* (1997), Simon & Schuster. (oh just read all SARK's books – they're so fabulous... especially Transformational Soup and this one!)

Ch. 5 Self-love is. . .

29. Ogden, J. & Evans, C. 'The Problem with Weighing: Effects on Mood, Self-esteem and Body Image' in *International Journal of Obesity 20* (1996), pp272–277.

Ch. 7 The What, When and How to of Eating

30. See http://www/usatoday.com/news/health/2006-11-15-slower-eating_x.htm
31. www.health.groups.yahoo.com/group/Mindoverfatter or e-mail: Mindoverfatter@yahoogroups.com
32. Email: info@ditch-diets-live-light.com
33. website: http://www.ditch-diets-live-light.com
34. website: http://www.mindoverfatter.co.za